Nutrition for Sport and Exercise

Nutrition for Sport and Exercise

Vincent Perkins

MURPHY & MOORE
www.murphy-moorepublishing.com

Nutrition for Sport and Exercise
Vincent Perkins
ISBN: 978-1-63987-405-7 (Hardback)

MURPHY & MOORE
Published by Murphy & Moore Publishing,
1 Rockefeller Plaza,
New York City, NY 10020, USA

Cataloging-in-Publication Data

Nutrition for sport and exercise / Vincent Perkins.
p. cm.
Includes bibliographical references and index.
ISBN 978-1-63987-405-7
1. Sports. 2. Exercise. 3. Nutrition. 4. Physical education and training.
5. Health. I. Perkins, Vincent.
GV703 .N88 2021
796--dc23

For more information regarding Murphy & Moore Publishing and its products, please visit the publisher's website www.murphy-moorepublishing.com

Table of Contents

Preface

The biochemical and physiological processes by which an organism makes use of food to support its life are studied under nutrition. These include ingestion, assimilation, biosynthesis, absorption and excretion. Sports and exercise bring changes in our muscular, neurohumoral and cardiovascular systems. These changes can affect our functional capacity and strength. Sport nutrition is the practice of diet and nutrition which aims to improve the athletic condition of human body. The nutrients studied within sport nutrition are classified into macronutrients and micronutrients. Carbohydrates, fats and proteins are categorized as macronutrients as they can be ingested in large quantities and are required for healthy cellular growth and metabolism. Important micronutrients for athletes include calcium, iron, zinc, vitamin B complex, vitamin C, D and E. Sport nutrition plays an important role in various strength and endurance sports such as cycling, weightlifting, bodybuilding, etc. The topics included in this book on nutrition for sport and exercise are of utmost significance and bound to provide incredible insights to readers. Some of the diverse topics covered herein address the varied branches that fall under this category. This book will provide comprehensive knowledge to the readers.

To facilitate a deeper understanding of the contents of this book a short introduction of every chapter is written below:

Chapter 1- Sports nutrition is a broad interdisciplinary field that focuses on the study and practice of nutrition and diet to improve the performance of athletes. It involves the application of nutrition knowledge to a practical daily eating plan to provide fuel for physical activity, facilitating the repair and rebuilding process after a physical activity and optimizing an athlete's performance. This chapter has been carefully written to provide an easy introduction to the varied facets of sports nutrition.

Chapter 2- Any physical activity requires good nutrition and hydration to provide energy. Every athlete has a unique energy requirement and their nutrition should be adapted as required. Energy need and energy intake should be monitored to provide energy balance. Energy and water needs of the athlete and other related topics are discussed extensively in this chapter.

Chapter 3- Dietary supplements are products taken orally as a supplement to a regular diet for the sole purpose of providing additional nutrients to the body. They usually contain one or more ingredients such as vitamins or amino acids. Energy bars, sports drinks, energy gels, diet drinks, etc. are all forms of dietary supplements. This chapter has been carefully written to provide an easy understanding of the subject matter.

Chapter 4- Weight management is the process of maintaining a healthy body weight through the combination of various techniques. Weight management plays an important role in sports where an athlete has to maintain a certain body weight and deliver a good performance at the same time. Overweight, underweight, weight gain, weight loss, calorie restriction, meal replacement, etc. are a few terms associated with weight management which are discussed in detail in this chapter.

Chapter 5- Doping or the use of performance enhancing drugs is a widespread phenomenon in sports. Performance enhancing drugs are substances used illicitly to improve athletic performance. This chapter sheds light on such practices and its side effects as well as the various measures, such as doping tests, taken to prevent it.

I would like to share the credit of this book with my editorial team who worked tirelessly on this book. I owe the completion of this book to the never-ending support of my family, who supported me throughout the project.

Vincent Perkins

1

The Basics of Sports Nutrition

Sports nutrition is a broad interdisciplinary field that focuses on the study and practice of nutrition and diet to improve the performance of athletes. It involves the application of nutrition knowledge to a practical daily eating plan to provide fuel for physical activity, facilitating the repair and rebuilding process after a physical activity and optimizing an athlete's performance. This chapter has been carefully written to provide an easy introduction to the varied facets of sports nutrition.

Sports nutrition is a topic of constant change and has grown as a dynamic field of clinical study. Research continues to advise improved nutritional guidelines and support for both active adults and competitive athletes. Science recognizes sports nutrition and energy intake as the "cornerstone of the athlete's diet." Sports nutrition is the foundation of athletic success. It is a well-designed nutrition plan that allows active adults and athletes to perform at their best.

It supplies the right food type, energy, nutrients, and fluids to keep the body well hydrated and functioning at peak levels. A sports nutrition diet may vary day to day, depending on specific energy demands. Sports nutrition is unique to each person and is planned according to individual goals.

The Goal of Sports Nutrition

Active adults and competitive athletes turn to sports nutrition to help them achieve their goals. Examples of individual goals could include gaining lean mass, improving body composition, or enhancing athletic performance.

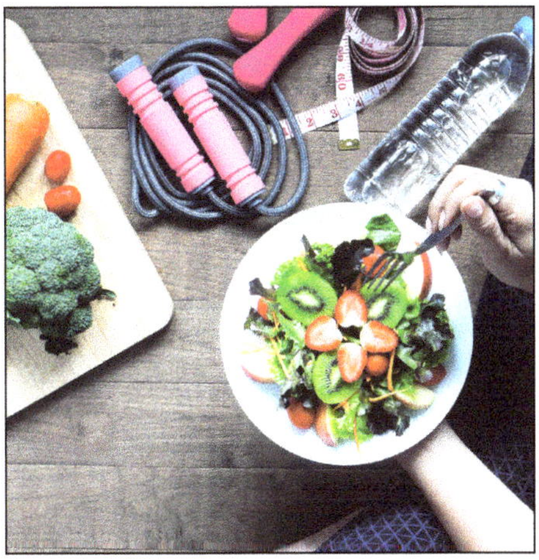

These sport-specific scenarios require different nutritional programs. Research findings indicate the right food type, caloric intake, nutrient timing, fluids, and supplementation are essential and specific to each individual. The following are different states of training and competitive sport benefiting from sports nutrition.

Eating for Exercise/Athletic Performance

Training programs require a well-designed diet for active adults and competitive athletes. Research shows a balanced nutrition plan should include sufficient calories and healthy macronutrients to optimize athletic performance.

The body will use carbohydrates or fats as the main energy source, depending on exercise intensity and duration. Inadequate caloric intake can impede athletic training and performance.

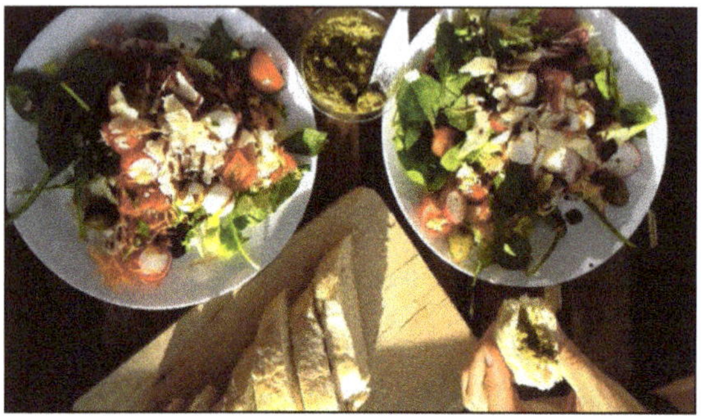

Active adults exercising three to four times weekly can usually meet nutritional needs through a normal healthy diet. Moderate to elite athletes performing intense training five to six times weekly will require significantly more nutrients to support energy demands:

- Carbohydrates are the main fuel source for an active adult or competitive athlete. General guidelines for carbohydrate intake are based on body size and training characteristics. Carbohydrate needs in a daily diet can range from 45 to 65% of total food intake depending on physical demands.
- Proteins are responsible for muscle growth and recovery in the active adult or athlete. Sufficient amounts of protein per individual help maintain a positive nitrogen balance in the body, which is vital to muscle tissue. Protein requirements can vary significantly ranging from .8g to 2g per kilogram of body weight per day.
- Fats help maintain energy balance, regulate hormones, and restore muscle tissue. Omega-3 and omega-6 are essential fatty acids that are especially important to a sports nutrition diet. Research findings recommend an athlete consume approximately 30% of their total daily caloric intake as a healthy fat.

Eating for Endurance

Endurance programs are defined as one to three hours per day of moderate to high-intensity exercise. High-energy intake in the form of carbohydrates is essential. According to research, target carbohydrate consumption for endurance athletes ranges from 6g to 10g per kilogram of body weight per day.

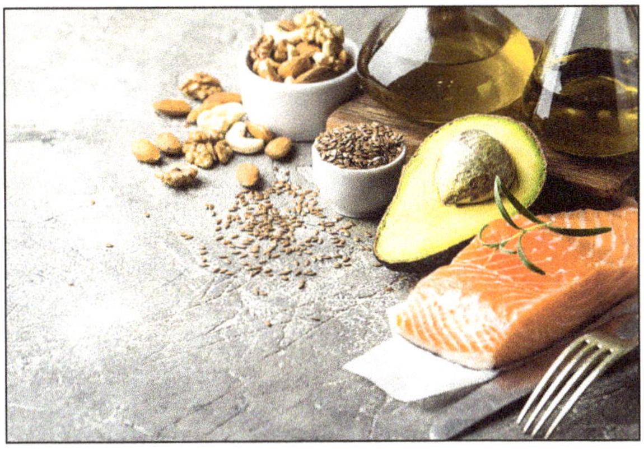

Fat is a secondary source of energy used during long-duration training sessions. Endurance athletes are more at risk for dehydration. Replacing fluids and electrolytes lost through sweat are necessary for peak performance.

Eating for Strength

Resistance training programs are designed to gradually build the strength of skeletal muscle. Strength training is high-intensity work. It requires sufficient amounts of all macronutrients for muscle development.

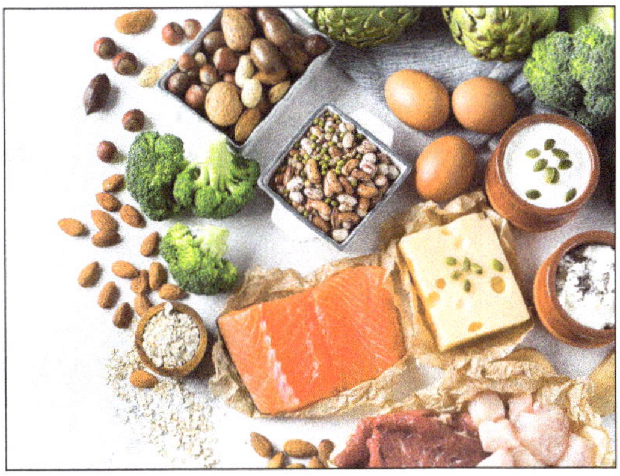

Protein intake is especially vital to increase and maintain lean body mass. Research indicates protein requirements can vary from 1.2g to 3.1g per kilogram of body weight per day.

Eating for Competition

Preparing for a competitive sport will vary in sports nutrition requirements. For example, strength athletes strive to increase lean mass and body size for their sport.

Endurance runners focus on reduced body weight/fat for peak body function during their event.

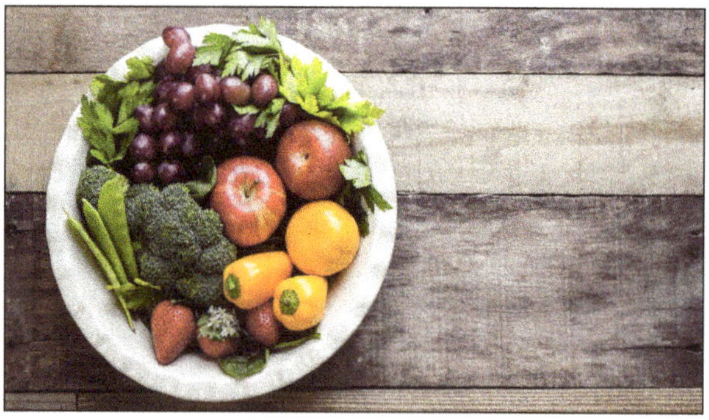

Athletic goals will determine the best sports nutrition strategy. Pre and post-workout meal planning are unique for each athlete and essential for optimal performance.

Hydration and Sports Performance

Adequate hydration and electrolytes are essential for health and athletic performance. We all lose water throughout the day, but active adults and athletes lose additional body water (and a significant amount of sodium) sweating during intense workouts.

Dehydration is the process of losing body water, and fluid deficits greater than 2 percent of body weight can compromise the athletic performance and cognitive function. Athletes are recommended to use fluid replacement strategies as part of their sports nutrition to maintain optimal body functioning.

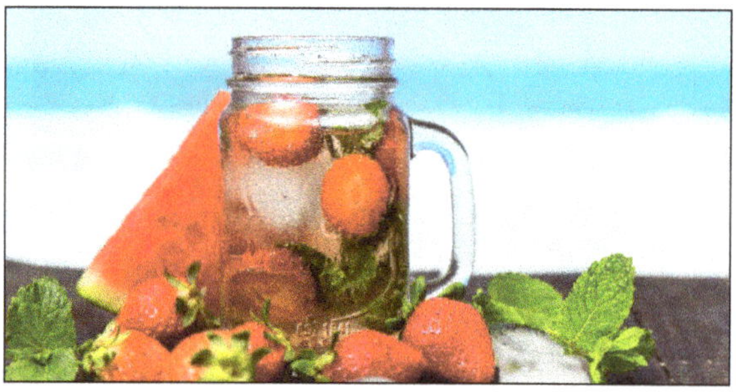

Rehydration with water and sports drinks containing sodium are often consumed depending on the athlete and sporting event. Lack of sufficient hydration for athletes may lead to the following:

- Hypohydration (dehydration),
- Hypovolemia (decreased plasma/blood volume),
- Hyponatremia (low blood sodium levels/water intoxication).

Supplements in Sports Nutrition

Sports supplements and foods are unregulated products marketed to enhance athletic performance. There are limited supplements backed by clinical research. The *Australian Institute of Sport* has provided a general guide ranking sports performance supplements and foods according to the significance of scientific evidence:

- Sports food: Sports drinks, bars, and gels, electrolyte supplements, protein supplements, liquid meal supplements.
- Medical supplements: Iron, calcium, vitamin D, multi-vitamin/mineral, omega-3 fatty acids.
- Performance supplements: Creatine, caffeine, sodium bicarbonate, beta-alanine, nitrate.

Special Circumstances

Sports nutrition covers a wide spectrum of needs for athletes. Certain populations and environments require additional guidelines and information to enhance athletic performance.

Vegetarian Athlete

A vegetarian diet contains high intakes of plant proteins, fruits, vegetables, whole grains, and nuts. It can be nutritionally adequate, but insufficient evidence exists on long-term vegetarianism and athletic performance. Dietary assessments are recommended to avoid deficiencies and to ensure adequate nutrients to support athletic demands.

High Altitude

Specialized training and nutrition are required for athletes training at high altitude. Increasing red blood cells to carry more oxygen is essential. Iron-rich foods are an important component of this athlete as well.

Increased risk of illness is indicated with chronic high altitude exposure. Foods high in antioxidants and protein are essential. Fluid requirements will vary per athlete, and hydration status should be individually monitored.

Hot Environments

Athletes competing in hot conditions are at greater risk of heat illness. Heat illness can have adverse health complications. Fluid and electrolyte balance is crucial for these athletes.

Hydration strategies are required to maintain peak performance while exercising in the heat.

Cold Environments

Primary concerns for athletes exercising in the cold are adequate hydration and body temperature. Leaner athletes are at higher risk of hypothermia. Modifying caloric and carbohydrate intake is important for this athlete. Appropriate foods and fluids that withstand cold temperatures will promote optimal athletic performance.

Eating Disorders and Deficiencies

Eating disorders in athletes are not uncommon. Many athletes are required to maintain lean bodies and low body weight and exhibit muscular development. Chronic competitive pressure can create psychological and physical stress of the athlete leading to disordered eating habits. Without proper counseling, adverse health effects may eventually develop. The most common eating disorders among athletes may include:

- Anorexia nervosa,
- Bulimia,
- Compulsive exercise disorder,
- Orthorexia.

Obviously, the nutritional needs of these individuals greatly differ from that of other active adults or athletes. Until someone with an eating disorder is considered well again, the primary focus should be put on treating and managing the eating disorder and consuming the nutrition needed to achieve and maintain good health, rather than athletic performance.

Micronutrient deficiencies are a concern for active adults and athletes. Exercise stresses important body functions where micronutrients are required. Additionally, athletes often restrict calories and certain food groups, which may potentially lead to deficiencies of essential micronutrients. Research indicates the most common micronutrient deficiencies include:

- Iron deficiency can impair muscle function and compromise athletic performance.
- Vitamin D deficiency can result in decreased bone strength and reduced muscle metabolic function.

- Calcium deficiency can impair the repair of bone tissue, decrease regulation of muscle contraction, and reduce nerve conduction.

Nutrients for Sports

Your body will require essential nutrients from food so that it can perform at its best. Failing to meet your nutritional requirements might leave you feeling lethargic, fatigued and failing to recover as quickly after training sessions and events.

Carbohydrates – Fuel for your Sport

Need of Carbohydrates

Carbohydrates get a bad rep with many people associating a high carbohydrate diet with weight gain. This is a myth and it is not the case if you choose your carbohydrates wisely. Think of carbohydrates as your source of energy or like putting petrol in a car. The more active you are, the more you will need to up your carbohydrate intake (exactly like how a car driven regularly needs to be refueled regularly). An active person who limits their carbohydrate intake may find that they don't have energy to perform at their best and may not recover quickly between sessions.

Including Carbohydrates in Diet

There are 2 main types of carbohydrates: fast and slow release. Both are useful in a diet to fuel sports, but timing is key:

- Aim to consume slow release carbohydrates throughout the day and fast release carbohydrates 1-2 hours before training and throughout training if you are taking part in >1-hour activity.
- During the day, aim to comprise a 1/3 of your main meals slow releasing carbohydrate - e.g. oats, Weetabix, brown pasta, brown rice, wholegrain bread or wraps, sweet potato or potato, couscous or quinoa.
- White versions will still give you the energy you need, but wholegrain versions tend to offer more health benefits.
- 1-2 hours before training, you might find it helpful to top up your energy stores by eating a light snack based on a carbohydrate e.g. toast and banana, fruit & granola and honey, dried fruit and nuts.
- After training, you can replace your stored energy (glycogen) by having a light snack or a meal containing carbohydrate. This means you will be ready to go for your next training session.

Protein – Promoting Muscle Recovery and Growth

Need of Protein

Protein is found naturally in many of the everyday foods that we eat, and if you are following a well-balanced diet, there should be no need to supplement. Protein is essential for repair and recovery of muscles and cells, so this is essential to prioritise in your diet if you are active.

Including Protein in Diet

- Aim to make 1/3 of your meals based around protein e.g. eggs, chicken, turkey, red meat, fish, tofu, legumes (beans, chickpeas, peas and lentils), cottage cheese, yoghurt, etc.
- 1-2 hours before your training, you might find it helpful add protein to your snack, e.g. cottage cheese, nuts, yoghurt, eggs.
- After training, you can promote recovery by having a light snack or meal containing protein.
- Don't panic if you can't eat straight after your workout. It is more important what you do overall in a day than what you do in the hour after working out.

Vitamins and Minerals – Keeping your Health at its Optimum

Need of Vitamins and Minerals

Your body requires vitamins and minerals to function at its best too. As your body can't make them, a well-balanced diet is essential to give your body what it needs. A deficiency can lead to feeling tired and run down. Nutrients of concern for athletes include iron, calcium, B vitamins and vitamin D. A quick blood test by your GP can signal if you are deficient in any of these key nutrients. In general, if you are eating for appetite and not restricting your food intake whilst eating a wide variety of foods you should be meeting your requirements.

Consumption of Enough Vitamins and Minerals

- Try to make 1/3 of your meals fruit or vegetables to ensure that your body is getting the nutrients that it requires. Soups, salads, roasted vegetables, smoothies, raw fruit and veg are all ways to reach your recommended intake. Aim to eat the rainbow and eat as many different types of fruits and veg as possible.
- Aim to consume milk, yoghurts or cheese 3-5 times a day depending on your age (children, teenagers and young adults need more while they are actively growing bones). These are excellent sources of calcium.

- Good sources of iron include red meat, chicken, turkey, eggs and legumes so if you are adding a good quality protein source to main meals you should be meeting your quota.

Fats – Increase the Healthy Fats and Decrease the Unhealthy Fats

Need of Healthy Fats

Healthy fats are so important to provide the body with fat soluble vitamins, energy and essential fatty acids. They are really important for mental health, as well as physical health.

Consumption of Enough Healthy Fats

- Although it can be tempting when you are active to “eat what you want”, try to limit processed foods like pizzas, doughnuts, cakes and biscuits which are not beneficial for sports or health.
- Healthy fats from oily fish (salmon, mackerel, herring) as well as nuts, seeds and avocados are beneficial in the diet in small amounts. Try snacking on a small handful of nuts with fruit or yoghurt, add seeds to your daily porridge or smoothie or top off a salad with half an avocado.
- Fats are energy rich though and can lead to weight gain if eaten in large quantities, so portion control is key here.

It is best to eat regularly throughout the day with a light snack 1-2 hours pre-training and post-training. This is to help prepare your body for action and recovery. Don’t stress out though if you miss a meal. The most important thing is that 80% of the time you are aiming to make healthy choices which will help to boost your performance.

Some Meal Ideas

- Porridge with yoghurt, nuts and mixed berries.
- Weetabix with milk and banana.
- Chicken sandwich with avocado and salad.
- Sweet potato with salmon and roasted vegetables.
- Chicken curry with rice and vegetables.
- Spaghetti bolognaise with pasta and vegetables.

Some Snack Ideas

- Pitta bread with cottage cheese and honey.
- Bagel with sliced fruit and natural nut butter.

- Chocolate milk and nuts.
- Smoothie made with milk and frozen fruit.

Nutrients for Endurance Athletes

Quite simply, athletes need more nutrients than less-active people. They demand more from their bodies than even average fitness buffs and so must compensate with the right nutrients from foods or supplements to keep performance—and recovery—at its peak.

The more intense the exercise or sport, the greater the body's nutrient needs. Athletes who participate in endurance sports—those that involve more than one hour of consistent activity—have specific needs because of what they demand from their bodies. For example, athletes lose more electrolytes, such as magnesium, potassium and sodium, through perspiration and must diligently replace them. The wear and tear of intense activity may necessitate increased intake of antioxidants such as vitamin E, which can help protect muscle cells from oxidative damage. Since muscle-tissue breakdown is common during intense exercise, athletes also need more proteins to repair the tissues. To keep their bodies performing optimally, endurance athletes should be familiar with these 10 important nutrients.

The first seven essential supplements are the minerals calcium, iron, magnesium, potassium, selenium, sodium and zinc. Their benefits range from keeping bones strong to minimizing fatigue.

1. Calcium: This may be the most important nutrient for an athlete. In a survey of more than 10,000 male and female athletes ages 7 to 50, fewer than half consumed 1,000 mg of calcium daily. The recommended dietary intake ranges from 1,000 to 1,500 mg/day depending on age and gender.

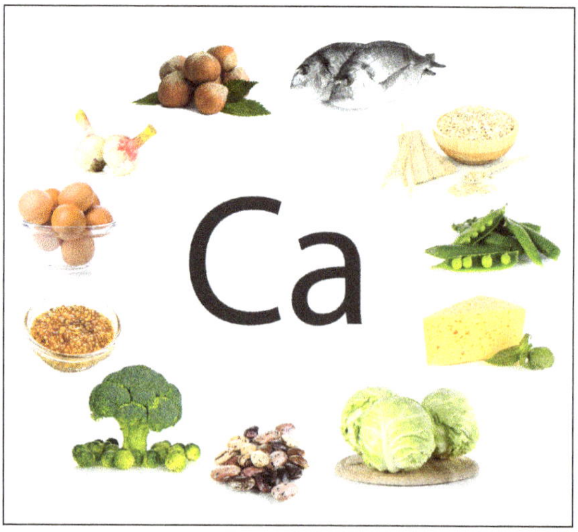

For female athletes, calcium intake is of particular concern. Excessive training—more than seven hours per week—may cause hormonal declines in young girls that can stop menstruation. This hormonal decline also compromises bone formation, possibly leading to premature, irreversible osteoporosis. Recent research shows that male endurance athletes of all ages experience testosterone deficits that also can cause osteoporosis.

Athletes Should monitor their calcium intake. Dairy foods can supply the required amounts unless sensitivities exclude them from the diet. But a diet without dairy foods requires supplements. All athletes should make sure they get 1,200 to 1,500 mg of calcium daily from food or supplements. Drinking a cup of skim milk, for example, provides about 300 mg of calcium.

2. Iron: For the casual athlete who trains less than four hours per week, iron deficiency is no more of a concern than for a sedentary person. But athletes who train for six or more hours per week often have iron-deficiency anemia and should be checked yearly for the condition. Female athletes who are unable to correct such mild anemia through diet can benefit from supplements.

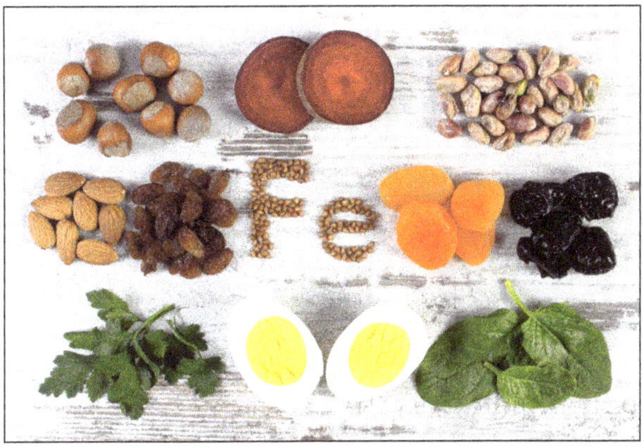

Athletes use iron stores more quickly than non-athletes and, considering the neurologic effects of anemia on children and teens who engage in rigorous sports, adequate intake of iron is quite important. The recommended dietary allowance (RDA) for iron ranges from 10 to 15 mg/day—an amount easily acquired from food. In the absence of anemia, athletes shouldn't take any supplemental iron because it raises the risk of heart disease and colon cancer.

3. Magnesium: This mineral is involved in adenosine triphosphate (ATP) production from fatty acid oxidation, post-contractile muscular relaxation, and bone remineralization. It is also involved in phosphatidylglycerol (DPG) production, which is important to red blood cell formation. ATP, present in all cells but particularly in muscle cells, stores energy. Low magnesium levels can acutely contribute to early fatigue, nausea and muscle cramps. Chronic magnesium deficiencies can lead to increased osteoporosis risk and anemia.

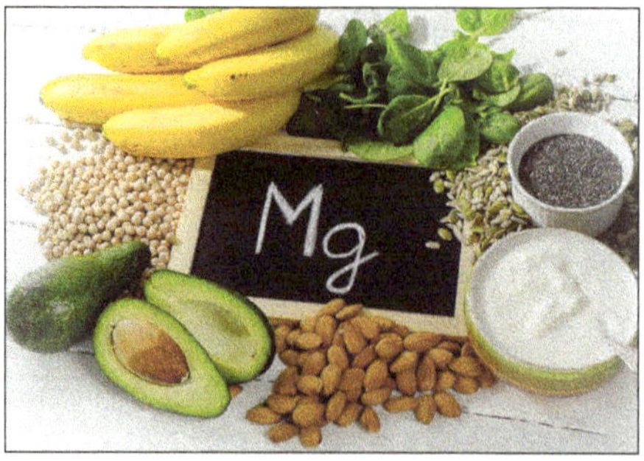

Athletes lose magnesium through sweat and urine. This, combined with the fact that athletes' diets are usually low in magnesium, generally leads to the need for supplementation. Recommended intake for endurance athletes is 500 to 800 mg daily. Higher doses can cause diarrhea.

4. Potassium: This mineral, present in intracellular fluid, is responsible for regulating total body water and stabilizing controlled and automatic muscle contractions. It is also lost through sweat and urine.

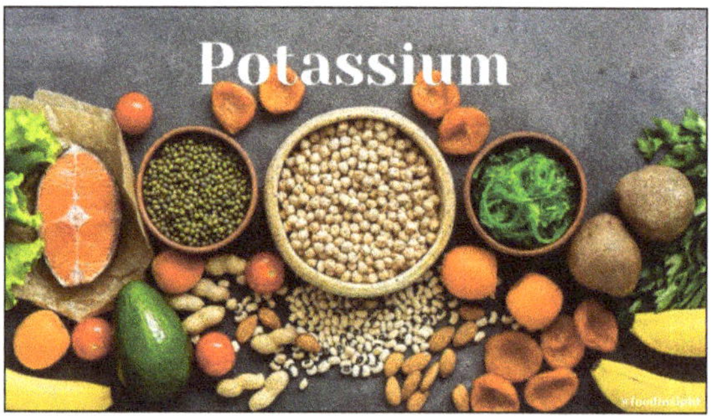

In a study of athletes running 40 minutes at 70 degrees Fahrenheit, potassium loss was estimated at 435 mg/hour. The rate of potassium loss is approximately 200 mg/kg of weight lost during exercise.

Cells release potassium into the bloodstream and serum levels rise with exercise, possibly instigating fatigue. Potassium supplementation after short events (less than two hours), and during and after long events, is warranted. For post activity replacement, athletes should take about 435 mg/hour of exercise or 200 mg/kg of weight loss. As much as 150 mg/hour during activity can be tolerated by most athletes. Supplement potassium cautiously because too much too quickly can cause cardiac arrest. Supplementing with potassium during training does increase markers of recovery, primarily serum lactate and muscle hydration, but does not aid performance.

5. Selenium: Essential to antioxidant glutathione peroxidase (SeGPx) production, selenium is a free radical-scavenging tripeptide made up of glutamine, cysteine and glycine. It is concentrated in the lining of the GI tract and lungs, in the liver, and in skeletal muscle.

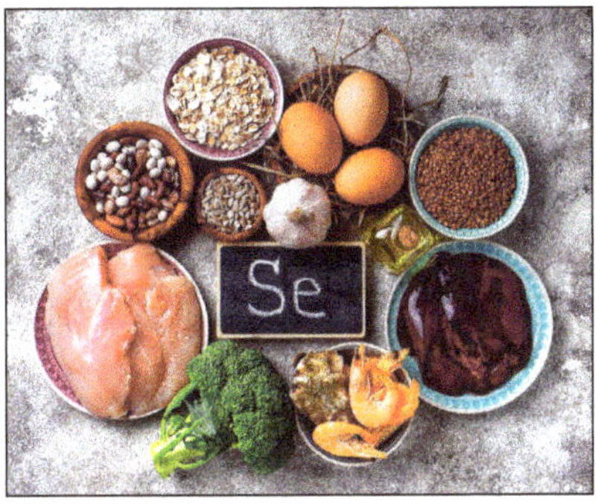

Research shows selenium benefits athletes' immune function and helps repair cellular damage. Researchers studied the selenium supplementation effects on muscle SeGPx in 24 healthy nonsmoking males. Half took 240 mcg of sodium selenite; half took placebo. After cycling to exhaustion—durations ranged from 2.6 to 3.5 hours—the group that took selenium showed less cellular damage. Supplementation with 200 mcg of selenium is safe and warranted for endurance athletes.

6. Sodium: This element helps cells retain water and prevents dehydration. Sodium also enables ATP generation. For events lasting longer than five hours, especially in hot weather, hypernatremia (dangerously low sodium) is a real concern. This especially applies to first-time or slower-running marathoners. Most organized events have aid stations with salty snacks. Anyone out for more than a few hours, especially on a warm day, should make sure to get some salt from snacks and fluid-replacement drinks.

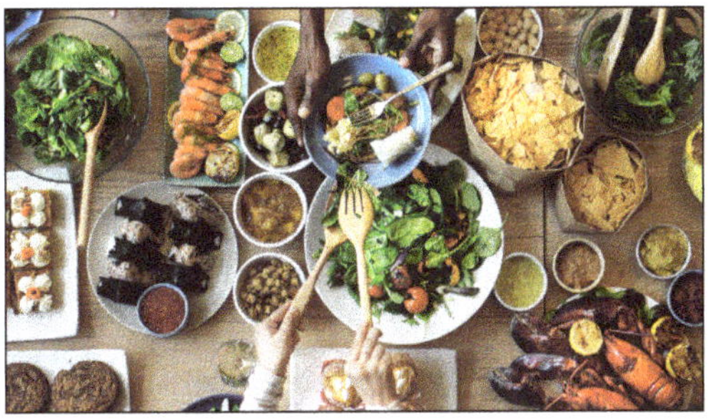

A prospective study was performed on 36 athletes during a three- to four-hour triathlon and 64 athletes at an ironman race, which lasts between nine and 15 hours. No athletes were hyponatremic after the shorter race, but 27 percent were hyponatremic following the ironman. An average of 17 percent of the ironman participants required medical attention, most for hypernatremia. Extrapolated from that study, athletes should aim for 80 to 100 mg sodium per quart of hydrating beverage and 100 to 300 mg sodium per hour from other sources.

7. Zinc: This mineral aids in post-exertion tissue repair and in the conversion of food to fuel. Both male and female athletes have lower serum zinc levels compared with sedentary individuals. Studies correlate endurance exercise with periods of compromised immunity—zinc depletion may be one reason.

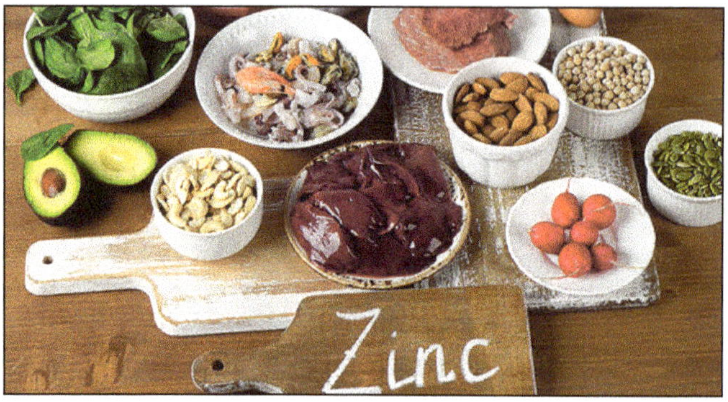

Those who train without days off lose zinc even more quickly. In a study of cyclists, researchers looked at zinc excretion via sweat. Half of the group underwent intense training for two months. Half underwent moderate training with two to three days off per week. Both groups were studied before and after. The exercising group showed increased zinc excretion while the control group showed no increase. The researchers believe altered zinc metabolism coupled with increased zinc excretion and stress levels lead to fatigue and decreased endurance. Athletes should take 30 to 60 mg zinc daily. Zinc picolinate or monomethionate are most easily tolerated.

Prevent Oxidative Damage

Antioxidants are another set of nutrients that endurance athletes are wise to use. Vitamin E: For athletes, one of the most important antioxidants is vitamin E. Aerobic athletes may have an increased need for this vitamin because their cells undergo more oxidative damage. Research shows athletes have less cellular damage when they ingest more vitamin E. Aerobic exercise places additional demands on the molecular free radical scavengers of the body, and vitamin E is a well-known scavenger.

In a study of 30 top-class cyclists, five months of supplementation with natural vitamin E (alpha-tocopherol) at an 800-IU daily dose significantly decreased markers of oxidative damage to muscle tissue. However, vitamin E did not benefit athletic performance.

Studies evaluating vitamin E as an ergogenic, or performance aid, show no benefit. One possible exception is at higher altitudes where oxidative stress is more intense. A group of six mountain climbers took 400 mg synthetic vitamin E (dl-alpha-tocopherol acetate). During exertion at altitude, they showed less output of pentane and lactic acid—both markers of oxidative damage, but not suggestive of improved athletic performance. The athletes also showed a statistically significant increase in anaerobic threshold compared to a placebo group.

The amount of vitamin E necessary to benefit athletes is not obtainable through diet. The jury is still out on natural vs. synthetic vitamin E, but endurance athletes should take 400 to 800 IU/day.

Protein and Glutamine

Without adequate protein and glutamine, athletes can feel the effects of reduced metabolism, poorer recovery times and increased susceptibility to infections.

1. Protein: The RDA for protein is 60 mg per day for adults (specifically 0.8 g/kg of body weight/day). This recommendation, however, is based on the needs of sedentary individuals. Recent studies indicate that protein needs increase during strenuous activity, which applies to both strength and endurance athletes.

Endurance athletes need more protein for different reasons than strength athletes do. Endurance athletes primarily use protein for maintaining aerobic metabolism, compared with the increased tissue-repair needs of strength athletes. When intake is inadequate, the body sequesters the needed proteins from lean tissue, which gives over trained endurance athletes a gaunt appearance. A protein deficit also impairs an athlete's recovery and wound-healing ability.

Researchers recommend endurance athletes eat 1.2 to 1.4 g/kg of body weight/day of protein. For a 155-pound athlete, this means a total of 85 to 100 g protein per day. Only a few studies recommend protein intake levels as high as 2 g/kg of body weight/day.

2. Glutamine: This amino acid increases the numbers of lymphocytes and macrophages. When glutamine levels are low these immune cells show depressed activity. Prolonged exercise consistently lowers glutamine levels. Glutamine supplementation reduces vulnerability to infections after prolonged exercise, though a few studies examining this phenomenon at lower exercise intensity levels have not shown benefit.

Oral glutamine replacement after exercise can lower infection risk. In one study, 200 runners and rowers were given placebo or 2,000 mg glutamine two hours after exercise. In the seven days following the exercise, 81 percent of the glutamine-supplemented group was infection-free compared to 49 percent in the placebo group.

A supplement that provides 2 g glutamine daily is a wise choice for athletes in training. Athletes who train strenuously for competition have greater nutritional needs than sedentary people. Adequate nutrients can mean quicker recovery time, lower infection rates, less fatigue, and ultimately, can help athletes reach their desired performance levels.

Dietary Assessment Methods for the Athlete

Investigating what an athlete eats is a daily activity for a sports dietitian, so it would be expected that the practice would make it an efficient and effective task. However, dietary assessment remains a challenge in sports nutrition, with the potential for significant errors of validity and reliability. These errors challenge the accuracy of estimates of what the athlete actually ate, or usually eats, and may also prevent the detection of a real change if an assessment is repeated. Developing expertise in this activity requires an appreciation that there are different reasons for undertaking an assessment, different approaches to completing it and different tools that can be employed. Therefore, the outcome can be enhanced by matching the best approach to each specific situation. Nevertheless, there is also a need to take into account the errors involved in a dietary assessment when interpreting the data that is collected.

Reasons for Collecting Dietary Information

Two basic scenarios explain why athletes might want to collect information about their food intake. In the first, the interest is in measuring what an athlete actually eats during a period in which they make their own choices. The chief goal of this activity, typically termed a dietary assessment, is to investigate what is happening without influencing the process. This scenario occurs in sports nutrition in a variety of situations of both research and athlete servicing, each with its own challenges and specific goals. Generally, dietary assessment methods are divided into strategies that are retrospective (what the athlete ate in the past) and those that are prospective (what happens over a period in the future). There have been four main methods used over the past 50 yrs to assess the dietary practices of athletes.

The second scenario, often known as diet tracking or self-monitoring, takes advantage of a limitation of many dietary assessment methods – that an individual will change his or her food intake during the process of monitoring it. A key tool in assisting an athlete to alter his or her dietary practices is to increase their self-awareness of their behaviour and the factors that underpin it. An athlete is likely to improve their food choices and portion control when they are accounting for their actions in real-time or directly associating their behaviour with an outcome. Receiving positive feedback about improvements in dietary practices and identifying the factors that support it can be valuable strategies in consolidating new habits. The protocols and tools used for dietary tracking activities may be different from those of dietary assessment because of the altered goals.

Retrospective Measurements of Dietary Intake

Retrospective methods include the dietary history (a guided interview usually used to gain insights on habitual intake, often framed as a typical day), the 24 h recall (which investigates intake over a specific day) and the food frequency questionnaire (a summary of usual intake of different categories of foods). A general principle common to each of these techniques is that they are heavily reliant on the athlete's ability to recall the types and quantities of foods and drinks consumed over the period of interest in the past. These methods fall short when the athlete is embarrassed/unwilling to reveal his/her true eating patterns or unable to provide good descriptions of the type and amount of items in his/her past intake. The 24 h recall is the least frequently used protocol, because situations in athlete practice or research in which we are only concerned about what happened on a single day are not as common as other interests. Food frequency questionnaires and dietary histories generally attempt to assess intake over longer periods of time, which is valuable in gaining a longer-term perspective on eating patterns. However, these techniques are reliant on the athlete's memory and insights into their true intake and suffer when the athlete is a poor historian and/or has a complicated lifestyle that is difficult to summarize.

The dietary history is commonly used by sports dietitians to gain initial insight into an athlete's dietary practices. Although it does not lend itself to an accurate quantitative assessment of nutrient intake, it is valuable for gaining insight into the pattern of meals, snacks, intake around training sessions/events and supplement use. It requires a skillful interview technique to gather information with minimal bias, to cross-check the information, and to probe for factors that contribute to the patterns of intake. Although it is challenged by the athlete's ability to accurately describe the usual portion sizes of their food and drink choices, the use of models or pictures of food sizes can assist the athlete to better describe the quantities they consume.

Food frequency questionnaires (FFQ) can be implemented by a trained interviewer, but can also be self-administered by the athlete, using paper or an electronic format, to save time and resources. Asking athletes to identify how often they eat a range of individual food/drink items may gain a summary of the total diet, but tends to overestimate intake in low-energy consumers and under-estimate intake in large eaters. Importantly, it strips away some of the information that sports dietitians are interested in – for example, when a food or drink is consumed and what else is consumed at the same time. Food frequency questionnaires are most useful to assess the intake of a particular nutrient or food factor of interest – e.g., antioxidants or calcium – where, ideally, the FFQ has been validated by comparing responses to a biomarker of the intake or nutritional status of the compound. Again, models or pictures of foods and portion sizes can help to enhance the accuracy of the identification or quantification of dietary intake.

Table: Traditionally used methods for collecting dietary intake information.

	Overview of Methods	Period of Interest	Pros	Cons
		Retrospective		
24 h recall	Subject describes foods consumed over the last 24 h or a "typical day.	24 h	Speedy to implement. Low burden for the subject. Interview can be structured around daily activities. Does not alter intake. Suited to epidemiological research.	Relies on subject's honesty, memory and food knowledge. Requires trained interviewer. Day for recall may be "a typical". Suitable for group surveys, but not representative of individual's normal intake.

Food Frequency Questionnaire (FFQ)	Subjects asked how often they eat foods from a standardized list and to estimate portion sizes often using photos or food models as a prompt.	From 24 h period to open-ended	Can be self-administered to lower burden on the investigator. Can be used to cross-check data obtained from other methods. Validated for ranking individuals. Can be modified to target certain nutrients. Can be automated to allow quick processing by investigator.	Relies on responder's honesty, memory, literacy and food knowledge. Validity dependent on the food list and the quantification method.
Diet history	Open-ended interview concerning food use, food preparation, portion sizes, food like/dislikes and a food checklist.	Open-ended or over a specified period	Accounts for daily variation in food intake by investigating a "typical" day. Can target contrasts between periods of interest as a subtheme. Collects information on timing of intake and factors that influence food patterns.	Relies on responder's honesty, memory, food knowledge. Labour intensive & time consuming. Requires trained interviewer. Mostly appropriate for qualitative assessment rather than quantitative.
Prospective				
Written food diary (diet record	Weighed	May be undertaken for 1-7 d, with increasing ability to track usual intake as duration increases, but reduced compliance	Provides a more accurate quantification of foods than household measures. Considered the "gold standard for dietary assessment".	Relies on participant's honesty and food knowledge. Time consuming for subjects to keep and investigator to process. Distorts food choice and quantity: Subject alters their diet to improve their intake or to reduce the workload of recording.
	Household measures (descriptions of cups, teaspoons, dimensions of food portions, etc.)		Improved compliance with subjects compared with weighed record. Less alteration of normal eating pattern compared to weighed or semi-weighed records.	See comments for weighed record. Requires checking by trained person. Needs standardized set of household measures. Subjective/ inaccurate assessment of portion sizes.

Prospective Measurements of Dietary Intake: The Food Diary

The food diary or diet record is the most popular dietary assessment protocol in sports nutrition research and practice. Having an athlete record what he/she consumes over a nominated period sounds like a simple task, but in reality, there is great complexity in making this exercise a meaningful one. Food diaries propose to monitor intake over a specific period that represents a generalized period of interest. This period may vary from a short-term dietary program (for example, the 48 h period prior to undertaking a research trial or a cyclist's intake during a multi-day stage race) to the athlete's typical diet. Variations on the traditional food diary technique include the number of days that are recorded and the method of quantifying food portions (e.g., direct weighing techniques or description via household measures and dimensions). Traditional paper and pen methods of recording place a large burden on the athlete and assume he or she is literate, motivated and organized enough to faithfully record their intake for the required period. There are several sources of error in prospective assessments:

- The athlete alters his/her eating patterns or food choices during the period of recording the food diary so that it does not reflect his/ her usual intake.
- The athlete records his/her dietary intake inaccurately to improve the perception of what he/she is eating (i.e., he/she omits or underestimates the intake of foods or meals seen as undesirable, or falsely reports the intake of foods seen as desirable).
- The athlete makes errors of quantification or description in recording his/her food intake.

Food diary protocols typically have trade-offs. For example, the weighed food record provides confidence in the accuracy of quantified information. However, having to weigh all food items – including individual components of a meal or dish – increases the burden on the athlete and usually leads to changes in food intake, whereby the athlete chooses foods that are simpler to process or skips the eating occasion entirely. Another trade-off is the duration of the food diary: An increase in the number of days of recording increases the likelihood that it represents the usual intake, but reduces the compliance shown by the subject in keeping an accurate record.

In the general population, a 3-4 d food diary is often considered the "middle ground" for investigating the intake of a group, but it is not often recognized that it provides a poor estimate of the true intake of individuals. Because we eat differently from day to day, there is considerable variability in our daily intake of energy and nutrients. Some dietary characteristics are stable, while other nutrients are less evenly distributed in foods, meaning that daily intakes fluctuate markedly and affect the precision of the estimate from a food diary. A study of the general population suggested that, 1) 14-30 d of records may be required to estimate an individual's intake of even the most stable nutrients to within 10% of their true long-term intake, 2) at least 7 d are needed to rank individuals within a group as high or low consumers, and 3) several orders of magnitude more are needed to accurately assess an individual's intake of variable nutrients. In addition, 4) having at least 15 subjects in a survey would allow a reasonable estimate of group average intake of stable nutrients (energy, carbohydrate) within 4-5 d of records, 5) moderately stable nutrients (e.g., iron) might require double the sample size or days recording, and 6) highly variable nutrients (e.g., vitamins A and C, cholesterol) could require >40 d or >200 subjects to derive a precise assessment. A practical way to gain a longer recording interval is to have groups or individuals keep several shorter records over a period of time, thus building up the total number of recorded days while reducing the drop-off in recording compliance.

Few studies have examined the optimal recording period for athletes by looking systematically at issues of recording compliance or day to day variability in food/nutrient intake. Professional experience suggests that some athletes are diligent – or even over-fastidious – at record keeping, accustomed to measuring aspects of their life in accurate detail and motivated by the idea that the activity could lead to better performance outcomes. Such individuals may be able to record a 7 d food diary with little burden and careful precision. Being able to monitor the duration of a training micro cycle is useful since it allows an assessment of how well patterns of food/fluid intake track with the changing needs of workouts and competition. Repeating such an assessment at different times of the periodized sporting calendar would build up a useful picture of the athlete's dietary practices. In contrast, other athletes are poor candidates for food diaries as an overcommitted lifestyle can leave little time or enthusiasm for real-time recording of food intake while the imposition by a coach of an effort-requiring activity when the athlete is disinterested in nutrition is unlikely to achieve a useful outcome.

Errors of Misreporting in Food Diaries

The different errors in food diaries affect the outputs in different ways. In some cases, the error involves inaccurate recording (the athlete ate food that he/she did not account for) while in others, the problem is atypical eating (the athlete ate the food, but it does not reflect his/her typical practices). Extensive study of the accuracy of food diaries in the general population has found that the bias of misreporting errors is towards under-reporting usual dietary intake. It was found that ~30% of respondents in dietary surveys significantly under-reported their true intake and that across studies; energy intake was under-reported by ~15%. Factors that seem to predict under-reporting in the general population include being a high-energy consumer, being overweight and/or being weight conscious.

While it is tempting to apply a correction factor across the board to the results of studies, this is inappropriate for individuals, since in any group survey there are likely to be individuals who significantly over-report energy intake, those who under-report and those whose reported intake is within reasonable agreement. Furthermore, there is evidence that even if the degree of misreporting of energy can be ascertained, it does not necessarily correlate with the misreporting of nutrient intake. Certain types of foods or eating occasions are more likely to be misreported than others, either due to the inconvenience of reporting (e.g., snacks), failure to recognize that they represent intake (e.g., foods and drinks consumed during exercise) or the desire to appear to eat better than in reality (e.g., reduction in high fat and sugary foods, increase in fruits and vegetables).

In general nutrition, researchers try to validate dietary survey methods or the collected data with three different approaches. They may compare the information that is collected against the results from another method, e.g., FFQ vs. a food diary. This is not entirely satisfactory since it generally involves comparing one set/type of errors against another. Comparison to an observation of actual intake is a possible validity exercise, but is complicated to achieve, particularly over the long term. A comparison to an independent marker of nutrient intake or status is generally the preferred method, with options including comparison of self-reported protein or sodium intake to urinary measures of nitrogen or sodium. Little research of this type has been undertaken on athletes.

The most common approach to checking the validity of a food diary is to compare energy intake against a theoretical or measured assessment of energy expenditure, taking changes in body composition to estimate energy surplus or deficit, and thus, a marker of under- or over-recording of usual/required intake. In research settings, energy expenditure can be measured in a metabolic chamber or, in free-living subjects, with doubly labeled water. Several sophisticated energy balance studies have been carried out on athletes and most have found discrepancies between reported energy intakes and energy requirements. Prediction equations and wearable tracking devices (e.g., Sense wear) offer another level of assessment of energy expenditure in both research and practical settings, although some caution is needed regarding their ability to accurately represent the energy cost of high-level athletic activities. Many researchers and practitioners adopt the Goldberg cut-off, which looks at a reported energy intake relative to measured or predicted basal metabolic rate to identify implausible habitual eating patterns and thus significant misreporting in a food record.

Errors in Quantitative Nutrient Analysis

Although researchers and practitioners often assess dietary intake data qualitatively, by examining patterns of food intake in light of recommended nutrition behaviours, the goal of many dietary assessment activities is to gain a quantitative assessment of energy and nutrient intake. The traditional achievement of this quantitative assessment involves interpretation by the investigator of the self-reported food data (e.g., the food diary), coding decisions and data entry into a computerized dietary analysis program. Such programs access a food composition database that varies in terms of the source of the food composition data, the number of foods that are included, the range of nutrients for which data are available and the method of analysis used in obtaining the nutrient data. Although computer dietary analysis programs are now widely available and easy to use, it is recommended that data entry and interpretation of dietary survey information remain the role of appropriately trained investigators using standardized techniques and cross-checking. This may help to eliminate errors and reduce the variability in decisions such as quantifying portions of foods described by subjects, and matching food descriptions to foods contained in the database. Of course, the availability and validity of food composition data in these analysis programs represents a major limitation at the end of the dietary assessment process.

New Technologies for Dietary Assessment

Traditional methods of dietary assessment were largely developed as "paper and pencil" activities although in some cases, like FFQs, there was an early evolution of questionnaires into electronic formats that could be filled out and assessed automatically. Such mechanization substantially reduces the burden both to the subject and the assessor. However, over the past decade, technological advances have allowed the evolution of a host of new options to replace written questionnaires and diaries. There is a wide selection of new ways in which food intake information can be collected and processed, harnessing the utility, portability and ubiquity of present day electronic gadgets. Many of these options provide variations on the food diary with features that are suited to dietary assessment and/or dietary tracking tasks. Studies are currently being conducted to identify how well the features of these technologies and techniques can enhance the process of gathering information on food practices of special populations including athletes. Although tempting to simply compare the outcomes to the results collected by another survey technique, it is hoped that studies will be undertaken to validate dietary data against better "ground truth" measures such as biomarkers or direct observations of food intake. It is likely that despite some of the potential or actual advantages of these new techniques, there will always be residual problems with gaining self-reported dietary information from any population.

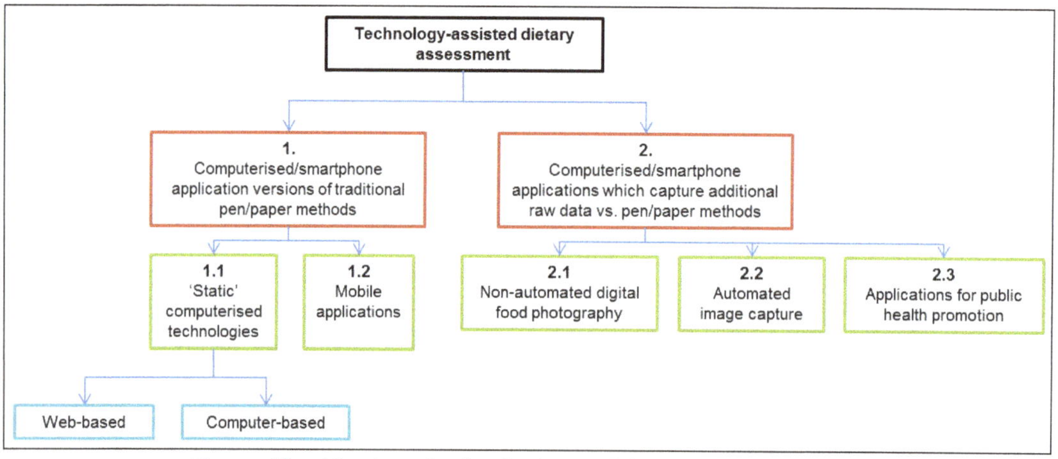

Figure: Classification of technologies used for dietary assessment.

Practical Implications

1. The following issues should be considered when choosing a dietary assessment method:

    - Validation: Has the technique been validated or explored in relation to athletes?

- Burden on the subject: How complicated, time consuming or intrusive are the demands?
- Characteristics of the subject: How literate, motivated and knowledgeable about food is he/she? What does he/she want to get out of the exercise?
- Burden on the researcher: How much time, expertise and resources are required to collect and process the information?
- Survey environment: What challenges are placed on the athlete during the assessment period? Will he/she be distracted or threatened by the information that is being collected?
- Features of interest: Are we interested in the intake of energy, macronutrients, micronutrients, other food chemicals, time of consumption over the day or in relation to exercise, or interaction of nutrients consumed at the same time?
- Assessment outcomes: Do we want quantitative, qualitative or ranking information?
- Are we interested in usual intake over a long period or specific intake over a short period?

2. Where prospective methods are used (e.g., food diaries), it is reasonable to expect that most athletes will under-record or under-consume their usual intakes:
    - Athletes who are weight/physique conscious or dissatisfied with their body image are at highest risk of significant under-reporting errors.
    - Best accuracy in self-reported dietary assessments might be expected from athletes who are confident of their eating habits and body image, and motivated to receive valuable feedback.
    - Training of subjects is likely to enhance their recordkeeping skills.
    - Processing of data from food records should be undertaken by qualified professional using standardized techniques.
    - Outputs from food diaries should be interpreted in light of under-reporting and misreporting issues, with checks of energy intake against measured or predicted energy expenditure providing information regarding misreporting.
3. New technologies and techniques of dietary assessment offer the advantages of in-

creased efficiency and lower subject/ researcher burden. However, validation of these techniques is required before we can be sure of their pros and cons.

4. The interpretation of self-reported information on dietary intake should be carefully filtered using insights about the dietary assessment tool and the athlete who used it.

2

Energy and Water Needs of Athletes

Any physical activity requires good nutrition and hydration to provide energy. Every athlete has a unique energy requirement and their nutrition should be adapted as required. Energy need and energy intake should be monitored to provide energy balance. Energy and water needs of the athlete and other related topics are discussed extensively in this chapter.

Energy Needs

Athletes rarely stay content with their progress for long, as a benchmark reached ultimately gives rise to another. They are in a constant strive to become stronger and faster, using the old adage "practice makes perfect" as a motivator to press forward. But no matter where a person falls on the athletic spectrum of recreational to elite, practice will only ever be half the battle. Poor or inadequate nutrition is often implicated in declining physical performance in athletes.

Science demonstrates how athletic performance changes based on nutritional intake. Athletes who reach and maintain peak performance are consistently the ones who best provide the requisite energy to fuel activity. These people are able to efficiently convert stored energy in to the power and endurance necessary for athletic success. In order to achieve this, athletes must be vigilant to not only consume the best types of calories, but also the correct amounts.

At its simplest physical level, the human form is basically a massive lump of stored energy. We eat energy, in the form of calories to fuel all of the functions that are necessary to live: respiration, circulation, movement, etc. This caloric demand increases proportionally with the number of calories expended in physical activity. Hence, athletes who tend to be very active, have a higher caloric need than the average person. To fully understand what is going on only requires a simple understanding of mathematics:

Calories Eaten – Calories Required = Net Calories.

When more calories are eaten than are required, net calories are positive, the extra calories are stored for future use as fat, and we gain weight. When fewer calories are eaten than are required, net calories are negative, our energy stores shrink, and we lose weight. Any severe imbalance, surplus or deficit, has metabolic implications that diminish athletic performance. The key to optimal athletic fuelling thus comes down to balance, where the net calories are effectively zero—that is, in a neutral state, where the number of calories eaten roughly matches the number of calories required.

Determination of the ideal caloric intake for individual athletes is very important. In general, a person is consuming the correct caloric intake if they have sufficient energy to compete in their sport without large fluctuations in weight. So long as a person avoids large magnitude deficits and surpluses in energy level, the metabolism appears to be able to self-regulate.

Existing in an energy neutral state may be ideal for an athlete at their desired body composition, but what about athletes who want to gain, or more commonly, lose weight? They must do so carefully, so to not impact athletic performance. Severe caloric restriction causes the metabolism to drop in order to preserve energy, which means that the body focuses on nutrient conservation and hinders energy usage in physical activity. When caloric restriction ends, the body reacts by storing calories, which ultimately results in rebound weight gain. Hence, severe calorie restriction not only impedes athletic performance, but also yields only temporary weight loss. Conversely, athletes who seek to gain weight by grossly over-consuming calories, no matter how rigorous their training schedule, risk decline in athletic performance by storing excess nutrients as fat rather than desired muscle. The key to modifying weight and body composition is to do so with no more than a 10-20% increase or decrease from their pre-determined energy neutral intake.

Athletes must consume enough energy, or calories, on a daily basis to meet their weight and body composition goals, whether it's to maintain weight, lose weight or gain weight. To maintain energy balance, the intake of solid food, liquids, and supplemental products must equal the energy expenditure.

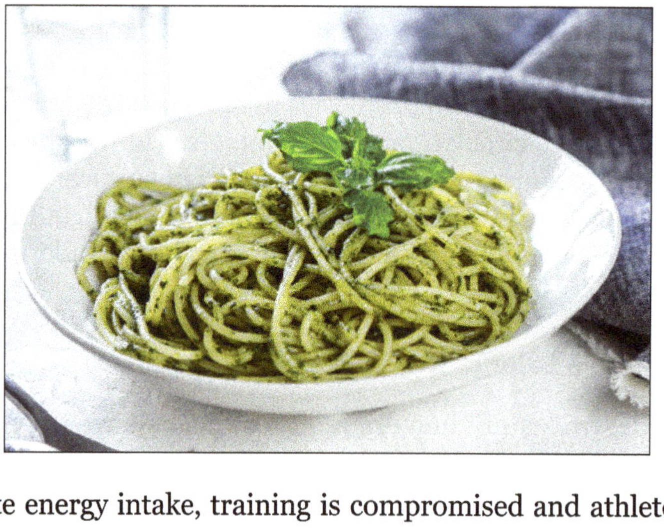

Without adequate energy intake, training is compromised and athletes are unable to meet their physical and performance goals. Loss of lean tissue can result, which can lead to hampered performance, often related to the loss of lean muscle mass or a decrease in endurance or power.

On the other hand, taking in too many calories can deter an athlete from reaching his or her body composition and performance goals. Extra calories form as fat in our bodies, and in most sports, an athlete's performance is enhanced with a body composition of primarily lean muscle and a low percentage of fat. Carrying around extra fat pounds will slow an athlete down.

There are several methods for calculating energy needs. A simple method is to take the athlete's weight (in pounds) multiplied by 10 for a rough average of basal needs, or basic needs without any exercise. Then, add in an activity factor and an average of calories burned for every minute of exercise. This is a very simplified way to get an initial calculation, from which to fine tune more specifically, but it gives a starting place.

For example:

> With a 220-pound athlete, calculate basal needs by multiplying the athlete's weight x 10: 220 x 10 = 2,200 calories.

For basic activity, multiply the calories by 20% to 30% and add it to the total:

> 2,200 x 1.2 – 1.3 = 2,640 – 2,860 calories.

Finally, to add exercise calories, add 100 calories for every 10 minutes of hard exercise or a workout. In this example, if the athlete trains hard for three hours on an average day (including sport-specific training and lifting/cross-training), an additional 1,800 calories.

> Total calorie needs = 2,640 – 2,860 calories + 1,800 calories = an average of 4,400 – 4,660 calories per day.

Step One

Calculate your basal metabolic rate (BMR), the minimal number of calories your body needs just for daily survival. Use this formula:

> BMR = 66 + (6.23 x weight in pounds) + (12.7 x height in inches) – (6.8 x age in years).

Example: If you weigh 220 pounds, you're 6′ tall, and 20 years old, your calculations would look like this:

> BMR = 66 + (6.23 x 220) + (12.7 x 72) — (6.8 x 20). That's 2214 calories per day.

Step Two

Calculate your Energy Expended for Physical Activity (EEPA), which is all the calories you expend in a day. You can figure this out with this formula:

EEPA = BMR x Activity Level.

Activity Level Factors

- 1.200 = Sedentary (little or no exercise due to injury or illness).
- 1.375 = Lightly active (about 30 minutes training, moderate 1 to 3 days/week).
- 1.550 = Moderately active (moderate 45 minutes, 3 to 5 days/week).
- 1.725 = Very active (1 hour, 6 to 7 days a week).
- 1.900+ = Extra active (very hard training including weight lifting 2-3 days/week).

Most athletes are between 1.550 and 1.9, depending on the training. For athletes training at very high levels (3 hours or more per day), calorie needs may exceed recommendations. Your EEPA based on 220 pounds and hard training is:

2214 x 1.9 = 4206 calories for BMR and EEPA.

Step Three

Calculate your Specific Dynamic Action of Food (SDA) by multiplying the total of BMR and EEPA in step two by 10%.

Example: Your SDA equals 4206 x 0.1 = 420 calories.

Step Four

Add the total from step two to the total from step 3 to get the overall number of calories you need daily to maintain your present weight.

Total Calorie Needs: *4206 + 420 = 4626 calories.*

Energy Intake and Expenditure

A regular supply of dietary energy is essential for life, and is required to fuel many different body processes. These include keeping the heart beating and organs functioning, maintenance of body temperature, muscle contraction and growth. However, daily energy requirements vary widely from one individual to the next. This is due to factors such as sex, body size, bodyweight, climate and physical activity levels.

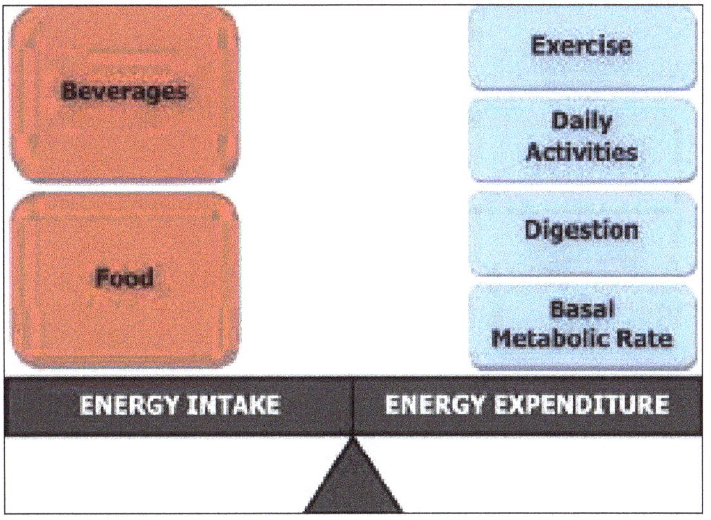

Energy is obtained, from the food and drink we consume, by oxidation of carbohydrate, fat, protein and alcohol, known as macronutrients. The amount of energy that each of these macronutrients provides varies:

- Fat is the most energy dense nutrient, and provides 9kcal (37kJ)/g.
- Alcohol is the second most energy dense nutrient, providing 7kcal (29KJ)/g.
- Protein provides 4kcal (17kJ)/g.
- Carbohydrate (starch and sugars) is the least energy dense nutrient, providing just 3.75kcal (16kJ)/g. [A value of 4 kcal is used for food labeling purposes].

Application of these factors to the food and drink consumed enables energy intake to be estimated. These days, energy intake is often measured in joules (J) (or kilojoules (kJ)) but many people are more familiar with Calories (kcal).

- 1 kilojoule (kJ) = 1,000 joules.
- 1 megajoule (MJ) = 1,000,000 joules.
- 1 kilocalorie (kcal) = 1,000 calories, or 1 Calorie.

To convert from one unit to another:

- 1 kcal = 4.184 kJ, so a 1000 kcal diet provides 4.184 MJ or 4184 kJ.
- 1 MJ = 239 kcal.

Energy expenditure is the sum of the basal metabolic rate (BMR) (the amount of energy expended while at rest at a neutral temperature and in the fasting state), the thermic effect of food (TEF) (otherwise known as dietary-induced thermogenesis) and the energy expended in movement of all types.

A substantial proportion of total energy expenditure is accounted for by BMR, which is determined principally by body mass and body composition both of which vary with age and sex.

Energy Requirements of Individuals

The actual amount of energy needed varies from person to person and depends on their basal metabolic rate (BMR) and how active they are.

Basal Metabolic Rate

The basal metabolic rate (BMR) is the rate at which a person uses energy to maintain the basic functions of the body – breathing, keeping warm, keeping the heart beating – when at complete rest. An average adult will use around 1.1kcal each minute just maintaining these functions and BMR differs from one person to the next, both within a population and between population groups. Infants and young children tend to have a proportionately high BMR for their size due to their rapid growth and development. Men usually have a higher BMR than women since they tend to have more muscle. Older adults usually have a lower BMR than younger people since their muscle mass tends to decrease with age. The BMR accounts on average for about three quarters of an individual's energy needs.

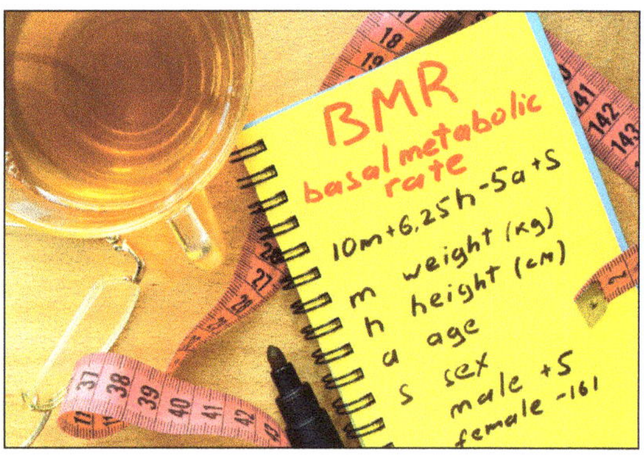
BMR
basal metabolic rate
10m+6.25h-5a+S
m weight (kg)
h height (cm)
a age
s sex
male +5
female -161

Physical Activity Level

In addition to their BMR, people also use energy for movement of all types. The amount of energy a person uses to perform daily tasks varies depending on factors such as his or her weight (the heavier a person is the more energy is required for movement) and their physical activity level. An estimate of the amount of energy an individual will need can be calculated by multiplying their BMR by a factor appropriate to the amount of activity that person does (known as the Physical Activity Level (PAL)). A PAL of 1.4 is associated with a very low level of physical activity at work or during leisure time. This applies to a large proportion of the UK population. In contrast, a PAL of 1.6 for women or 1.7 for men represents moderate intensity activity, and values of 1.8 for women or 1.9 for men represent high levels of physical activity.

Energy Expenditure = BMR x Physical Activity Level (PAL)

Using this approach and published data, estimates of average energy requirement for different population groups have been established.

Physical Activity

Physical activity should be an important component of our daily energy expenditure. Many different types of activity contribute to our total physical activity, all of which form an integral part of everyday life. Total physical activity includes occupational activity, household chores, care giving, leisure-time activity, transport (walking or cycling to work) and sport. Physical activity can further be categorised in terms of the frequency, duration and intensity of the activity.

Physical Activity Recommendations

Physical activity levels in the UK are generally low and of concern in virtually all sections of the adult population and among older children and teenagers. It is estimated that up to a third of boys and between a third and a half of girls are not sufficiently active. Only 35% of men and 24% of women meet physical activity recommendations.

In order to benefit health, individuals should undertake at least 30 minutes of at least moderate intensity activity on five or more days a week. Moderate intensity activity is defined as a level of activity that will:

- Lead to an increase in breathing rate.
- Lead to an increase in heart rate (the pulse can be felt during this level of activity).
- Lead to a feeling of increased warmth, possibly accompanied by sweating.

This does not have to be taken all at once – three brisk walks of 10 minutes duration would be equally beneficial. Also, more benefit will be gained if the activity extends beyond the 30 minute guideline.

These recommendations also apply to older adults, and in addition older people should aim to maintain mobility through daily activity; activities that promote and improve balance, strength and co-ordination are particularly encouraged.

Children and young people are recommended to engage in at least 60 minutes of at least moderate intensity exercise every day. Activities that increase muscle strength and flexibility and also improve bone strength (i.e. weight bearing activities that strengthen the skeleton) should be included at least twice a week. In order to prevent obesity, many individuals will need to participate in between 45 and 60 minutes of moderate intensity physical activity each day.

Estimated Average Requirements (EARs) for Energy throughout the Life Course

Tables below show the estimated average requirements (EARs) for energy for the UK population.

Table: Estimated Average Requirements for energy (children and adolescents aged 0-18 years).

Age	EAR MJ (kcal)/day Boys	EAR MJ (kcal)/day Girls
0-3 months	2.28 (545)	2.16 (515)
3-6 months	2.89 (645)	2.69 (645)
7-9 months	3.44 (8250	3.20 (765)
10-12 moths	3.85 (920)	3.61 (865)
1-3 years	5.15 (1230)	4.86 (1165)
4-6 years	7.16 (1715)	6.46 (15450
7-10 years	8.24 (1970)	7.28 (1740)
10-14 years	9.27 (2220)	7.72 (1845)
15-18 years	11.5 (2755)	8.83 (2110)

Table: Estimated Average Requirements for energy for groups of men and women with low activity levels.

	EAR	
Weight (kg)	MJ/day	Kcal/day
	MEN	
19-4974	10.6	2550
50-5974	10.6	2550
60-6474	9.93	2380
65-7471	9.71	2330
75+ 69	8.77	2100
	WOMEN	
19-4960	8.1	1940
50-5963	8.0	1940
60-6463.5	7.96	1900
65-7463	7.96	1900
75+ 60	7.61	1810

EARs for an individual vary throughout the life course. During infancy and childhood, it is essential that energy is sufficient to meet requirements for growth, which is rapid during some stages of childhood. Energy requirements tend to increase up to the age of 15-18 years. On average, boys have slightly higher requirements than girls and this persists throughout adulthood, being linked to body size and muscle mass. After the age of about 18 years, energy requirements tend to decrease but remain linked with the individual's level of activity. After the age of 50 years, energy requirements are estimated to decrease further in women in particular and after age 60 years in men, which is partly due to a reduction in the basal metabolic rate (BMR), as well as a reduced level of activity and an assumed reduction in body weight.

Intake Versus Expenditure

In order for people to maintain their body weight, their energy intake must equal their energy expenditure. Failure to maintain energy balance will result in weight change. Energy balance can be maintained by regulating energy intake (through the diet), energy expenditure (adjusting physical activity level to match intake) or a combination of both. Failure to compensate for an increase in energy intake with an increase in expenditure will result in weight gain (positive energy balance); conversely a reduction in energy intake which isn't matched by a reduction in physical activity levels will result in weight loss (negative energy balance).

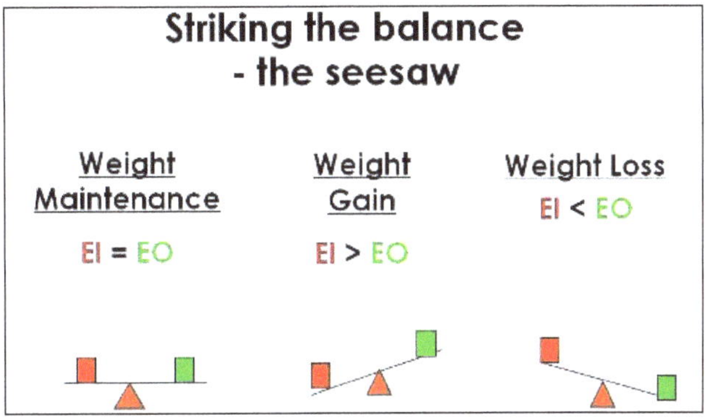

The average daily energy intake of UK adults is 9720 kJ (2313 kcal) for men and 6870 kJ (1632 kcal) for women. The sources of energy in the UK diet are shown in figure. These figures are below the EARs shown in Table below, for both men and women and have been falling steadily, year on year, for some time. At the same time, the population has become ever more sedentary and population obesity levels are still on the increase. Assuming the estimates of intake are correct, this means that energy expenditure levels have fallen to a greater extent than the reduction in dietary energy intake. This emphasizes the need for people to become more active because as energy intake falls, the greater is the likelihood that micronutrient needs will no longer be met.

The easiest way to increase physical activity level is to incorporate more activity into daily routines, e.g. walking or cycling instead of driving short distances, and taking up more active hobbies such as gardening or rambling. Within the workplace there are fewer opportunities for increasing activity levels, but stairs can be used instead of the lift and people can walk to speak to colleagues rather than using the phone or email.

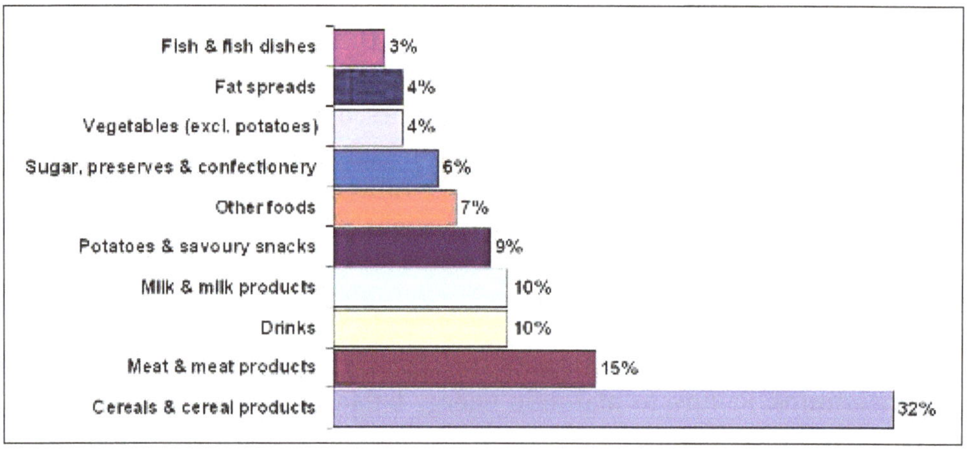

Below are some examples of the amount of energy expended over a period of 30 minutes for a selection of activities:

Physical activity	Calories used in 30 minutes
Ironing	69
Cleaning and dusting	75
Walking	99
Vacuum cleaning	105
Golf	129
Tennis (doubles)	150
Brisk walking	150
Mowing the lawn (using a power-mower)	165
Cycling	180
Aerobics	195
Swimming	195
Tennis (singles)	240
Running (10 minutes/mile)	300
Running (8.5 minutes/mile)	345
Running (7.5 minutes/mile)	405

Metabolic Pathway and Sport Performance

All biochemical pathways or processes are based on the utilization of one single molecule, ATP (Adenosine Tri-Phosphate), from bacteria to humans. ATP is a nucleotide in which the base adenine is linked to a sugar ribose, itself connected to three inorganic phosphate

(Pi). ATP is the only compound that, directly or indirectly, when hydrolysed, transfers chemical energy to all other processes that require energy, such as muscle contraction.

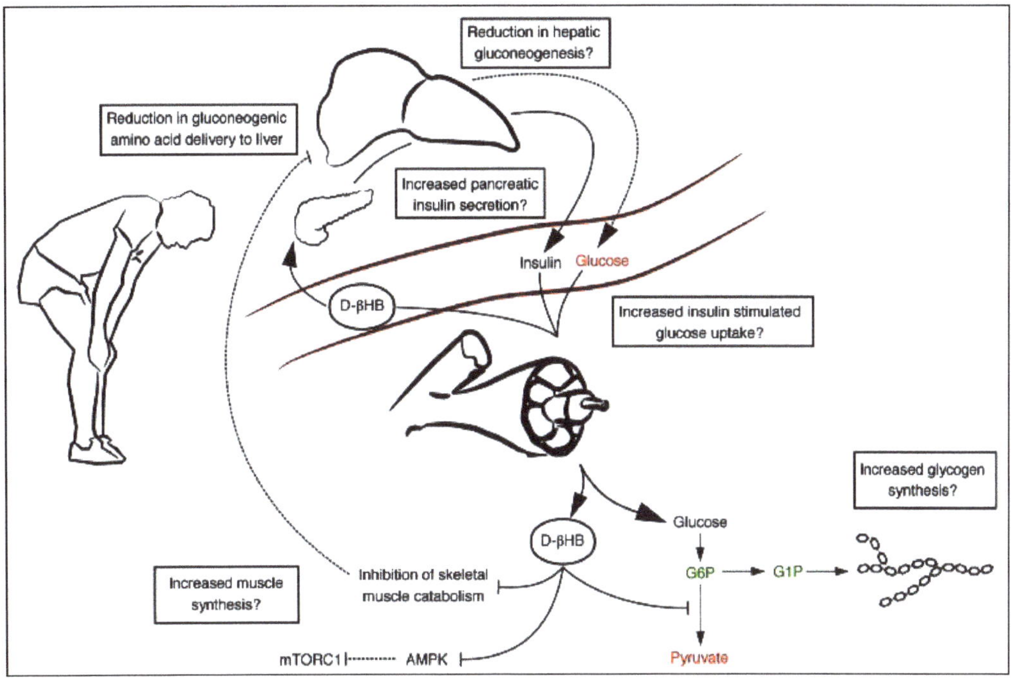

The development of biochemical tools (such as tissue biopsies and gene access), including molecular biology, has given access to the understanding of basic facts related to single muscle performance and adaptations during training schedules. However, knowing thermodynamic principles do not necessarily provide information about the rate at which a reaction will proceed. Enzymology is central to biochemistry but one has to know the limit of thermodynamic and kinetic principles of numerous enzymes and more precisely factors that change the activity of an enzyme. Moreover, the use of recent molecular biology techniques, such as the use of mRNA determination of an enzyme molecule, does not necessarily predict its synthesis. Additionally, some enzymes are "regulatory enzymes" that activate or inhibit the activity of a metabolic pathway, and thus the maximal activity obtained from that pathway. Unfortunately, some publications, even with high level of impact factors, do not take care of the limitations imposed by enzyme kinetics.

General Metabolic Pathways During Exercise

To perform muscle fibre contraction, there is a need for energy released from one single molecule, ATP converted to ADP (adenosine diphosphate) and Pi (inorganic phosphate). However, the total quantity of ATP molecules in human skeletal muscle is very low (5-6 mmoles/kg) and the energy demand for muscle contraction would be sufficient to sustain intensive shortening for only 2-3 seconds. Thus, a variety of fuels that lead to generation of ATP from ADP and Pi are needed to replenish this local tiny store. Besides ATP store, the striated muscle has also an almost immediate energy supplier called phosphorylcreatine (PC: 15-20 mmoles/kg) which transfers its phosphate group to ADP, replenishing therefore the ATP molecule during or after muscle contraction. However, this PC store would maintain theoretically heavy muscle contraction for another few seconds (< 7 s): not enough to beat the actual World 100 m dash! It appears therefore that other energy fuels are needed to sustain muscle activities during sport events.

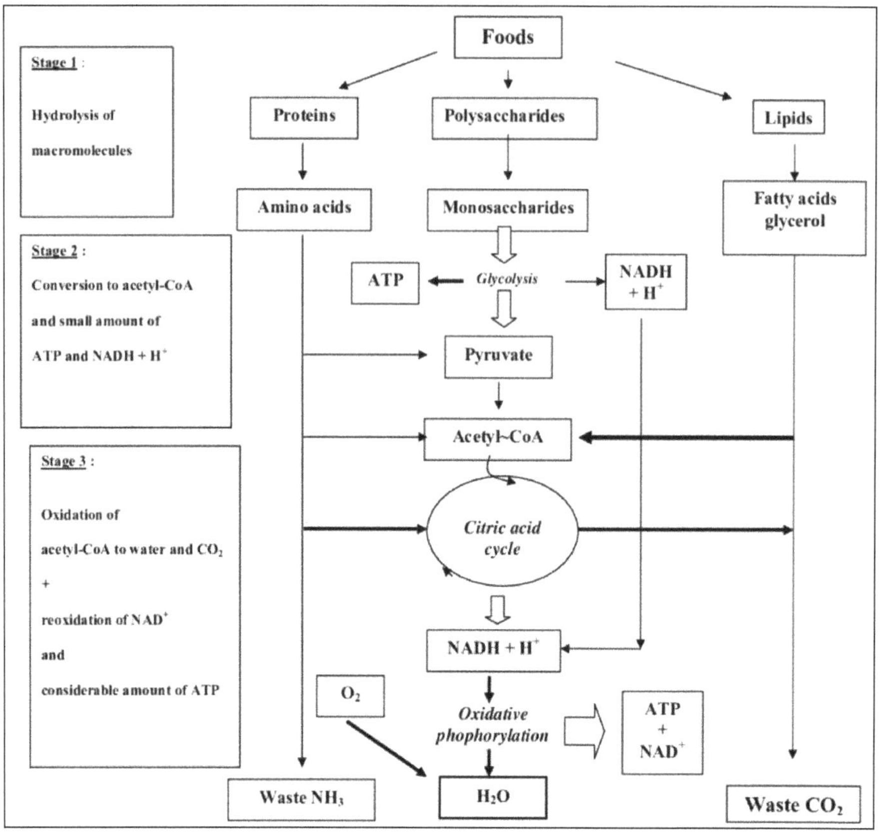

Figure: Illustrates the origin of ATP generation from food feeding and local human reserves (muscles, liver, and adipose tissue).

Catabolic reactions from food supplies and body reserves (muscles, liver, adipose tissues). Original macromolecules are hydrolyzed to single constituents giving rise to acetyl ~ and a few molecules of ATP and protons (H^+ and NADH) in the cytosol. Mitochondria (mainly) contributes heavily to the release of 2-3 carbon molecules from the three food substances to enter the Citric Acid Cycle (Hans A "Krebs Cycle") to produce more reduced cofactors (NADH and $FADH_2$) and H^+. On the inner surface of the inner mitochondria the protons enter into the sequence of electron transfer complexes in the chain of oxidative phosphorylation where most ATP synthesis will be produced from ADP and Pi molecules. The remaining body waste products are expelled by respiration (CO_2) and urine (NH_3, urea) to satisfy other living organisms.

Stage 1

Polymer molecules (proteins, carbohydrates, lipids) are converted to elementary substrates (amino acids, monosaccharides, fatty acids and glycerol). Those hydrolyzed reactions do not liberate energy immediately used by the muscle cells.

Stage 2

The monomere substrates are converted to simple molecules of three (pyruvate) or two (acetate) carbon, giving a few supplies of free energy molecules as ATP as well as reduced molecules (NADH, Nicotinamide Adenine Dinucleotide reduced-H).

Stage 3

All previous small molecules are converted to acetyl-CoA (acetyl-coenzyme A), then to a variety of metabolic pathways (such as the citric acid cycle, the ß-oxidation reaction) which release reduced molecules, NADH, $FADH_2$ (Flavine Adenine Dinucleotide reduced -H). The latter two molecules react with free oxygen (O_2) in the mitochondria giving enough energy to recombine ADP and Pi to ATP molecules. In human skeletal muscle (such as the vastus lateralis of the quadriceps), the ATP and PC levels are low, as compared to the local stores of macromolecules.

Moreover, in the whole organism, the available stores of energetic substances are diversely distributed. It appears that glycogen molecules are mainly located in skeletal muscles and liver, while triglycerides are stored in adipose tissues (visceral organs mainly). Additionally one has taken into account the maximal energy released from each type of substrates.

It appears that the maximal power released from muscle contraction comes from the few ATP itself which is very rapidly restored the other reserve stores. The energy release from ATP hydrolysis is thus obtained from direct small reserves of ATP and PC stores within the muscle fibres, then using the glycolytic pathway down to pyruvate ending by the oxidation pathways. Newsholme et al. estimated that the energy release from the glycolytic pathway (also called anaerobic glycolysis) amounts to 97-98% for a 100 m-dash, nearly 50% during an 800 m-run, and about 3% for a 5,000 m distance run. Hochachka and Somero gave a schematic estimation of metabolic rate (expressed as % of maximum) from the different substrates towards the intensity of the exercise. Eventually, the estimation of the metabolic fluxes releasing energy within a skeletal muscle fibre depends in fact upon two main factors:

- The availability of the energy stores (muscle and periphery).
- The maximal activity of the specific enzymes.

Besides the compulsory need of metabolic compounds, the catalysis of the various energy substances is absolutely connected to specific organic molecules acting at physiological temperature: Enzymes.

Table: Distribution of energy stores in the human vastus lateralis.

Substrates	Fresh tissue ($\mu mol.g^{-1}$)	Energy content ($kJ.mol^{-1}$)	Disposable energy ($\mu mol \sim P.g^{-1}$)
ATP	6	44	5.1 (1)
PC	15	58	9.9 (2)
Glycogen (glucose residue)	121	2,900	4,350
Triglycerides (ex. Palmitate)	9	29,300	3,510
Amino acids (free)	36	1,870	800

(1) = 90% ATP, ADP and AMP.
(2) = 67% PC, Creatine.

Table: Total energy stores in male human subject (70 kg body weight, 28 kg muscle mass, 15% fat mass), in the prandial phase.

Substrates	Total dry weight (kg)	Disposable energy (kJ)
Triglycerides	10.5	338,500
Proteins	6	78,250
Glycogen		
Liver	0.100	1,700
Muscles	0.500	8,500
Blood (glucose, fatty acids)	0.023	420
PC	0.087	17
ATP	0.076	5

Table: Estimation of power released from the different energy stores within a human muscle.

Substrates	Final products	Maximal power output ~ P ($\mu mol.g^{-1}.s^{-1}$)
ATP	ADP	3.00
PC	Creatine	1.60
Glycogen	Pyruvate, lactate	1.00
Glycogen	CO_2, H_2O	0.50
Free fatty acids	CO_2, H_2O	0.24
Amino acids	CO_2, H_2O	?

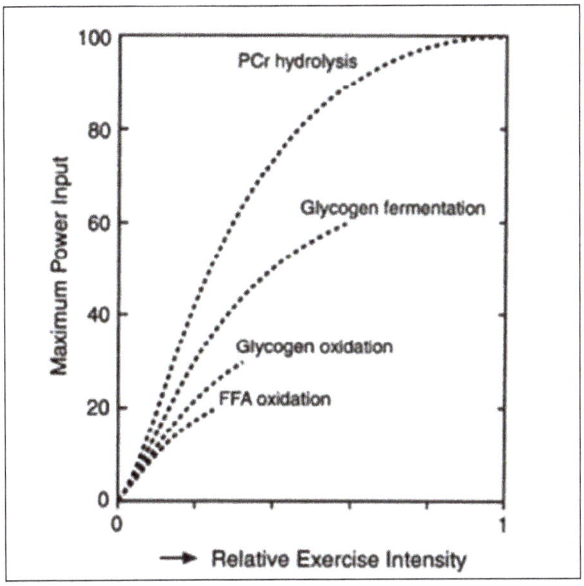

Figure: Relationship between fuels, major pathways, and maximum metabolic rate during exercise of progressive intensity.

Regulation of Enzyme Activities

All reactions, but one (creatine to creatinine), in the human body are under enzyme activities that proceed at a satisfactory rate in the cell. Enzymes are protein molecules (one or several molecules) having a catalytic action inside their structure. This active side is a three-dimensional structure that binds the substrate to the enzyme complex, which results in catalysis. The enzyme-substrate complex, which involves weak bonds, is readily reversed. The enzyme-substrate complex formation occurs if the substrate has groups of atoms that are in the correct three-dimensional orientation to interact with the binding atoms in the active site. Concentrations of substrates, temperature, protons (pH of the milieu) change the catalytic activity of an enzyme.

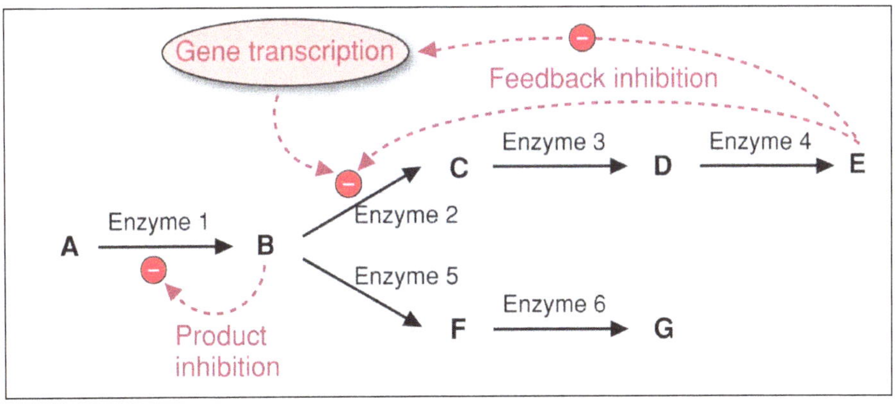

The catalytic activity of an enzyme is measured by the rate of its reaction proportional to the concentration of the enzyme. It varies according to the substrate concentration through a hyperbolic curve from first order (the activity increases approximately linearly with the increase in substrate concentration) to zero order (the substrate concentration has very little effect on the rate of reaction. However, the activity of some enzymes shows a sigmoid curve indicating that the activity of that enzyme can be either reduced or activated by small molecules (ligands) at the same concentration of the substrate. The latter type of enzyme belongs to an "allosteric" model of a better physiological significance. Indeed, the allosteric enzymes belong to the "substrate cycle system" of reversible reactions where the A to B reaction led by one enzyme is reversed by reaction B to A by another enzyme. The maximal catalytic activity (V_{max}) of an enzyme and its half Vmax (maximal velocity), expressed by the Michaelis-Menten constant (Km), has a physiological significance which can estimate the metabolic flux of a series of reactions.

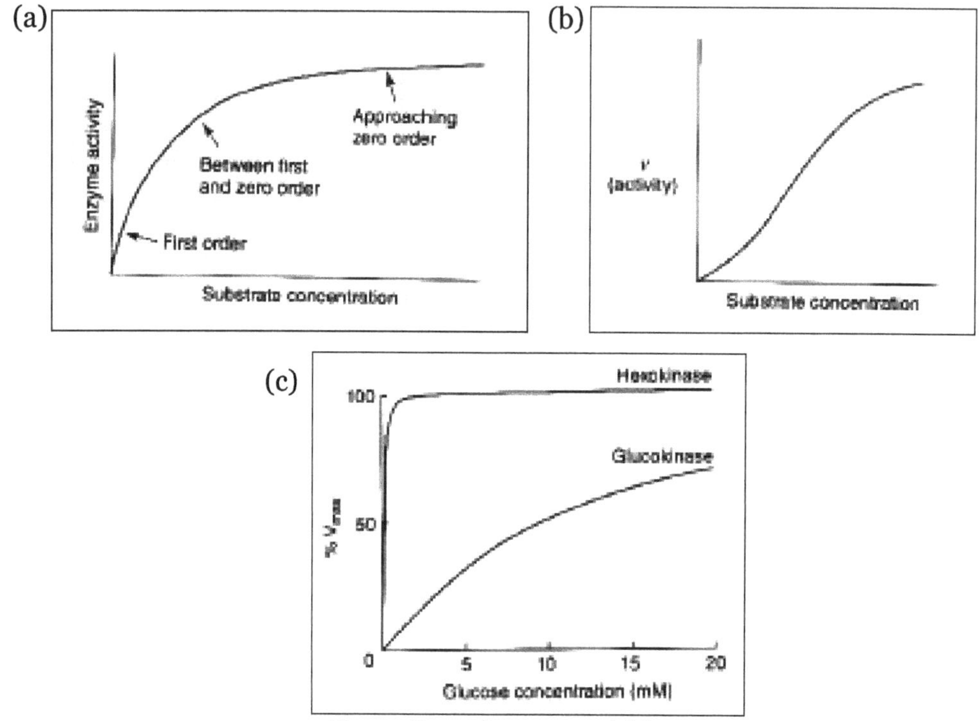

Figure: General enzyme activities.

(a) First and zero order components of hyperbolic curve of enzyme activity against substrate concentration.

(b) Sigmoid response of enzyme activity against substrate increase showing a greater inhibitory effect at lower concentration. The numbers represent the effect on the maximum activity of the enzyme, as compared to figure.

(c) Percentage of maximum activity of hexokinase and glucokinase against glucose concentration released specifically to muscle and liver. The difference of curves emphasizes a faster saturation of the enzyme in muscle tissue as compared to hepatocytes.

The Km value also provides information about the role of similar regulatory enzyme systems in different cells, such as the first step of glucose reaction in the glycolytic pathway (glucose to glucose-6-phosphate, G6P). In skeletal muscle, the hexokinase action has a very-low Km, meaning the enzyme is rapidly saturated by its substrate; in liver, the first step by glucokinase is never saturated by higher physiological concentration. Thus, figure demonstrates that muscle glucose uptake is rapidly saturated by normal concentration of arterial glucose, while liver can rapidly phosphorylate this sugar to be converted to glycogen stores after a meal.

Another value has a fundamental importance in understanding the relationship between biochemical pathways: the Gibbs free energy concept which combines the first and second laws of thermodynamics. Gibbs, an American scientist, used the definition of enthalpy (the heat produced by a reaction) together with the entropy (molecular disorder induced by the reaction) to determine the direction of a reaction of biochemical pathway:

$$A \rightleftarrows B$$

$\Delta G^o = - 2.3$ RT log Keq (1 mole concentration of B and A)

$\Delta G = \Delta G^o + 2.3$ RT log Γ (Γ = real concentration of B and A)

$\Delta G = - 2.3$ RT log Keq/Γ

Practically, the previous enzymatic properties means that one has to take into account the Km of each enzyme involved in the regulatory flux of the pathways, together with the inhibitor and stimulating actors of a precise substrate cycle. This approach is compulsory to understand the several hundred-fold increase of the glycolytic flux as soon as one is facing high intensive exercise.

Besides the free energy concept, one has also to consider the coupling of biochemical reactions. A two-substance reaction A $\rightarrow$ B can be coupled-in-parallel with another reaction X $\rightarrow$ Y by one specific enzyme E1. However, in many cases, the X molecule is regenerated through another couple C $\rightarrow$ D by another specific enzyme E2. Under those conditions we need to know the precise metabolic flux (in Joules or kcal) of these irreversible reactions (to evaluate the predominance of the real flux between the two reactions J1 and J2).

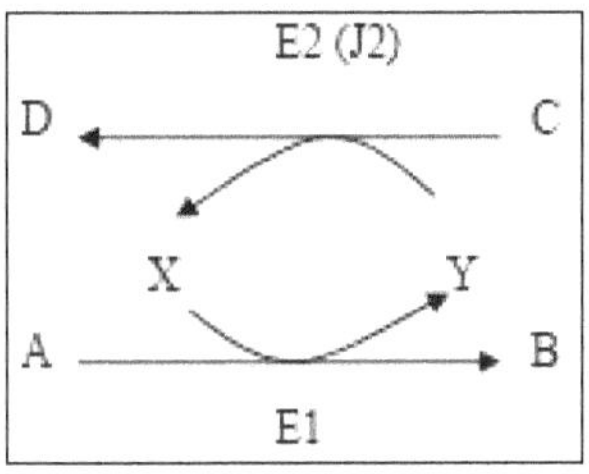

One example may clarify this concept: the substrate cycle between fructose-6-phosphate (F6P) and fructose-1,6-bisphosphate (F-1,6-BP) in muscle glycolysis under resting condition. The numbers express the metabolic flux J (µmol^{-1} kg.min^{-1}) in the human vastus lateralis.

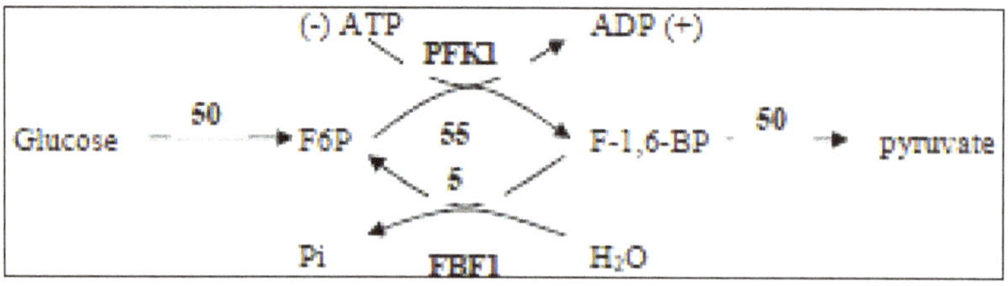

The enzyme phosphofructokinase 1 (PFK1) is inhibited by a resting level in ATP, while it will be activated by an excess of ADP released under heavy exercise. It may be already visualized that the synthesis to glucose from pyruvate is a much slower process. This observation points out another important fact related to kinetic reaction within a substrate cycle. We may consider the existence of equilibrium and non-equilibrium reactions within a substrate cycle. When there is a maximum catalytic activity for one enzyme as compared to a much lower activity for the other enzyme, this situation characterizes a non-equilibrium process. Conversely, a reaction is near-equilibrium if the activities of the two enzymes are close to each other. Thus in the above example of PFK1, we are facing a far-from equilibrium reaction, the enzyme activity being moderate with a high ATP/ADP ratio (resting condition), or at full maximal activity under a low ATP/ADP ratio (exercise condition).

Metabolic Regulation of Carbohydrates

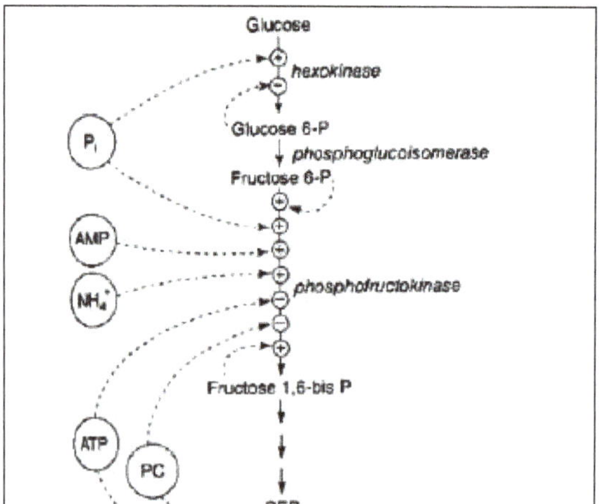

Figure: Factors involved in regulation of keys steps in glycolysis.

Glycogenolysis and glycolysis within skeletal muscle fibres are regulated by far-from equilibrium enzymes. Glucose taken up by blood supply (from liver glycogen) is catabolized by 10 enzyme reactions down to pyruvate. Only three substrate cycles induced by far-from equilibrium enzyme systems are involved in the regulation of the glycolytic flux from glucose to pyruvate. Those enzymes are either activated or inhibited by small molecules (ligands) involved in local metabolism, such as ATP, ADP, AMP, Pi, and PC.

Three regulatory enzymes lead the way glycolysis down to pyruvate. Small molecules will act to stimulate (ADP, AMP, Pi, NH_4^+,) or reduce (ATP, PC,) glycolysis according to the need to enhance, or not, the synthesis of new molecules of ATP for muscle contraction, as an example.

In order to shed light of these regulatory couples, one has to analyze the free energy status of enzymes involved in striated muscle glycolysis. All three enzymes leading to the production of pyruvate from glucose are far from equilibrium. Moreover, muscle glycogen degradation to glucose molecules is led by another substrate cycle that involves glycogen phosphorylase and glycogen synthase.

Phosphorylation of the two enzymes by ATP and a specific protein kinase has opposite action on glycogen molecule. Doing so during exercise, the release of one glucose molecule is favoured, while glycogen synthesis is inhibited, the two enzymes being next to glycogen molecules.

The entrance of pyruvate into mitochondria is the next step under enzyme regulation. The oxidation and decarboxylation of pyruvate by pyruvate dehydrogenase (PDH) and its NAD cofactor releases acetyl-CoA and NADH + H^+. Indeed, under resting condition, the PDH action is slow down by the available concentration of ATP. Then, the acetyl-CoA enters the citric acid cycle (CAC, also call the Krebs cycle) were molecules of NADH, $FADH_2$, H^+ are released (as co-enzymes) using specific enzymes.

Again, the flux of the CAC is led by three allosteric enzyme systems (out of a total of 8 enzymes), all far from equilibrium. These enzymes are activated or inhibited by their co-factors being in excess, such as ATP, NADH, ADP, Ca^{2+}, ...Citrate synthase (CS), isocitrate dehydrogenase (ICDH) and oxoglutarate dehydrogenase (2-OGDH) are the key enzymes regulating the flux of the CAC by non-equilibrium reactions. However, the limiting flux of the cycle is under the leadership of the lowest activity member, 2-OGDH. This explains why the oxidative flux of CAC (unit of metabolite.g $tissue^{-1}$.min^{-1}) is much lower than that obtained by glycolysis.

From those experimental observations, one has to choose the correct enzyme system to understand why there is no anarchy within a resting muscle. When there is no need to produce new ATP molecules in the oxidative phosphorylation system (such at rest), the regulatory enzymes slow down the activation of the glycolytic and mitochondrial pathways, favoring the synthesis of carbohydrates (and fat weight while overeating and keeping out of exercise.

Enzymes	ΔG° Kj.mol-1	Keq	Γ	Keq/ Γ	ΔG° Kj.mol-1	Equilibrium
Hexokinase	-20.9	4,700	0.08	59,000	-27.9	far from
Phosphof-ructokinase	-17.1	1050	0.03	35,000	-26.5	far from
Aldolase	+23.0	1.10^{-4}	9.10^{-5}	11	-6.1	near
Pyruvate kinase	-24.7	2,000	40	-15.8	-15.8	far from

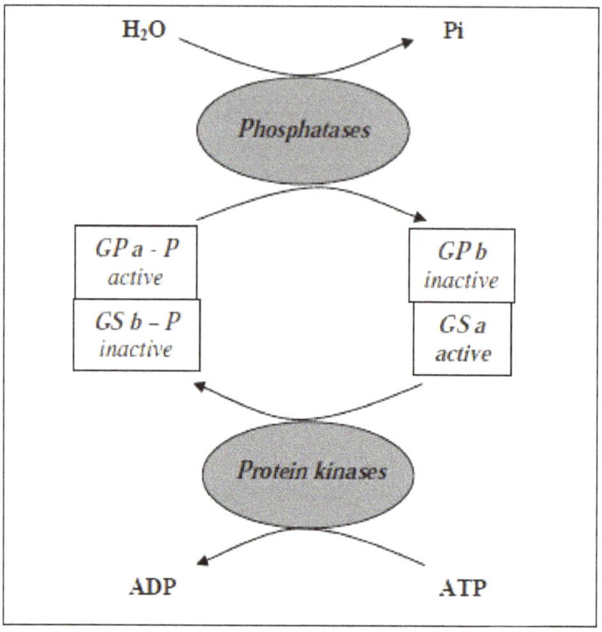

Figure: Mechanism of adaptation of glycogen degradation or synthesis in muscle and liver tissue according to the demand of energy. All enzymes are closed to the glycogen granules located in the cytosol.

When there is a need of excess energy, such as during exercise, glycogen release molecules release glucose to enter glycolysis. Proteins kinases stimulate the phosphorylation of glycogen phosphorylase a (GP-a), which become active, while inhibiting glycogen synthase b (GSb). Thus, the release of glucose molecules is stimulated to enhance the production of ATP molecules in sarcoplasmic and mitochondrial sites. After exercise, the reverse situation occurs to refill the glycogen store. Again, the concentration of small molecules (ATP, ADP), together with specific hormone stimuli (adrenaline), appear to lead the compulsory need to replenish the less content of energy stores: ATP.

Phosphorylation of PDH inhibits the enzyme (PDHb) whereas phosphorylation activates the enzyme (PDHa). Increase in Ca^{2+}, ADP, NADH concentrations is thus the main stimuli to foster the activity of the Citric Acid Cycle, and thereafter the production of new ATP molecules.

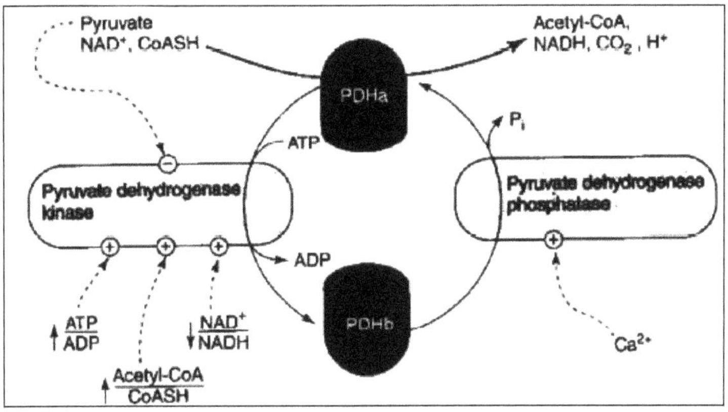

Figure: Regulation of the activity of pyruvate dehydrogenase (PDH) by small molecules from metabolic cycles.

Intense exercise enhances the amount of Ca^{2+} within the mitochondria amplifying the activity of ICDH and 2-OGDH, together with the increase of ADP content.

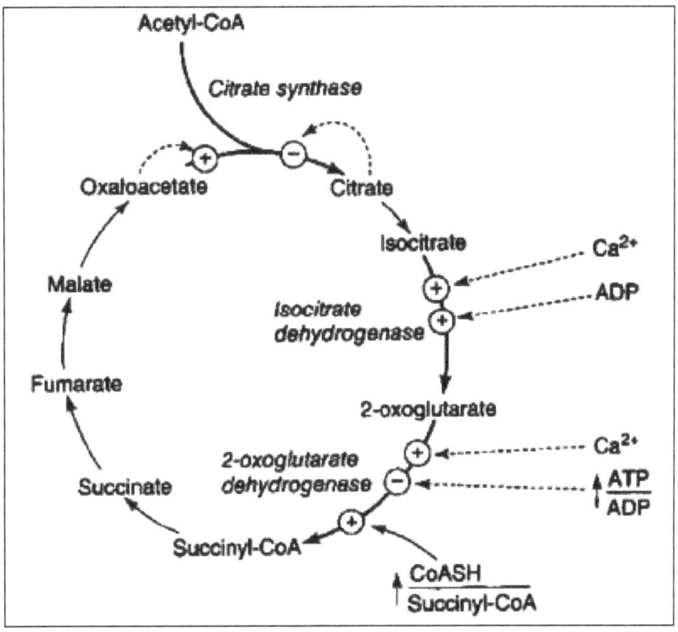

Figure: Control of the metabolic flux of the CAC during physical exercise.

Metabolic Regulation of Fatty Acids

The next regulation to investigate, as far as the limitation factor is concerned, is the transfer of free fatty acids into the mitochondria. The fatty acid has to be linked to coenzyme A (CoA) in the cytoplasm, forming a fatty acid-CoA molecule which is transported across the external membrane of the mitochondria to react with carnitine (an amino acid derivative synthesized in the liver and the kidney) by a specific enzyme, the fatty acid-carnitine. Taking an example with a C16 fatty acid molecule (palmitate), the enzyme is called carnitine palmitoyltransferase 1 (CPT1).

Carnitine palmitoyl transferases (CPTI and II) are located on the outer (CPTI) and inner (CPTII) surface of the inner side of the inner membrane of the mitochondria. They are reacting with all longchain fatty acid. The incorporation of free fatty acids to the matrix of mitochondria and their access to the CAC are thus limited by the maximal activity of the CPTI and II.

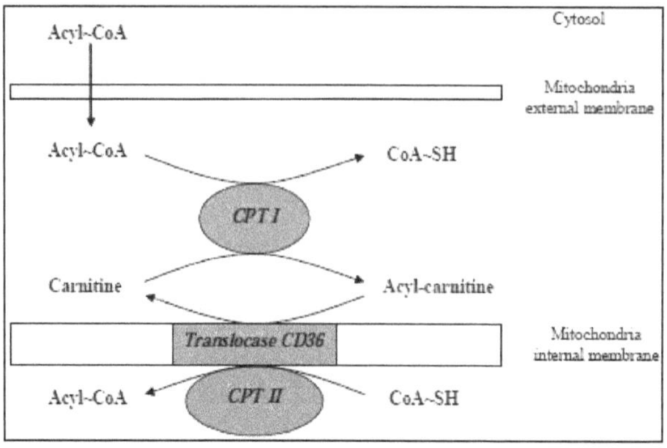

Figure: Transport of long-chain fatty acid molecules across the inner mitochondrial membrane.

A translocase transfers the fatty acid-carnitine complex through the inner membrane of mitochondria and another fatty acid-carnitine complex (herewith CPT2) liberates the fatty acid to the matrix of the mitochondria where each fatty acid will enter the so-called ß-oxidation pathway (each long-chain fatty acid is oxidized step by step releasing acetyl-CoA molecules which enter into the Krebs cycle). The limitation step of fatty acid oxidation is the carnitine acyltransferase complex having a low Km, and thus a rapid saturated flux.

Metabolic Adaptations During Exercise in Human Subjects

The effect of different types of running on contents of glycogen (muscle and liver) and muscle concentrations of ATP, ADP, PC, Pi and lactate have been measured to evaluate, indirectly, the stimulation of specific metabolic pathways:

Table: Effect of running exercise on muscle glycolysis in human subjects.

Activities	Glycogen (% from rest)	ATP $\mu M.g^{-1}$	PC $\mu M.g^{-1}$	Pi $\mu M.g^{-1}$	Lactate $\mu M.g^{-1}$	ATP/ADP ratio
Rest	100	6.2	22.0	1.0	0.75	60
400 m	85	5.2	1.9	27.0	23.00	5
2 km	81	5.0	4.2	22.0	28.00	5
21 km	11	5.7	7.2	25.0	3.50	5

It appears that short sprinting lowers PC concentration but has a reduced effect on glycogen stores. On the contrary, long distance endurance running depleted mostly glycogen content but has a moderate depletion in PC store and lactate production. In all exercise conditions, the muscle ATP store remains relatively high, but the Pi shows a major increase while the estimated ATP/ADP ratio drops to 10% as compared to resting condition. Thus, it seems quite clear that small ligands, such as Pi, ADP leads to the activation of specific regulatory enzymes.

How could we investigate the metabolic adaptation related to any modification of a specific pathway (being activated, or not), as evidence of a change in enzyme activity? The answers are: 1) to choose the right limiting enzyme in a metabolic cycle; 2) to measure the quantity of that enzyme. The latter investigation implies the isolation of that enzyme knowing that the metabolic flux is directly related to the amount of enzyme available in that tissue. At first glance, as soon as we do identify the limiting enzyme, we have to apply the general mechanism of protein synthesis through the usual sequence: DNA → mRNA → protein synthesis. For many years, molecular biologists did apply this sequence using highly specific tools. Nevertheless, we now know that mRNA amplifications do not implicitly postulate that new molecules of enzymes (proteins) have been made up in a tissue. Moreover, the last decade gave us new tools to investigate biogenesis in skeletal muscle: The discovery of microRNA (miRNA) that posttranscriptionally regulates the expression of target genes. The miRNAs are a class of about 22 nucleotide in all animals, plants and unicellular eukaryotes non-coding RNAs that control diverse biological functions. DNA proportion from miRNA molecules represent about 60% of the total DNA package within a cell, while DNA leading to protein synthesis is near to 2% of the whole DNA particles. Over 1000 miRNAs have been identified within the human genome, and a single miRNA may inhibit several target genes, thus acting on skeletal muscle differentiation, such as during skeletal myogenesis. The increased production of miRNA will slow down the synthesis of new protein molecules by inducing mRNA cleavage, either by translational inhibition and or by promoting the degradation of target mRNA, thus inhibiting the production of new protein molecules.

For certain, miRNAs are playing a major role in explaining adaptations to cardiac and skeletal muscle hypertrophy in resistance exercise training, in sarcopenia. Apparently, results from plasma circulating miRNAs might have potential value as physiological mediators of exercise-induced cardiovascular adaptation in athletes. Looking to the effects of exercise training, it becomes clear one needs to choose the correct enzymes to evaluate changes of specific metabolic adaptations in skeletal and cardiac muscles.

Energy Balance

"Energy balance" is the relationship between "energy in" (food calories taken into the body through food and drink) and "energy out" (calories being used in the body for our daily energy requirements).

This relationship, which is defined by the laws of thermodynamics, dictates whether weight is lost, gained, or remains the same. According to these laws, energy is never really created and it's never really destroyed. Rather, energy is transferred between entities.

We convert potential energy that's stored within our food (measured in Calories or kcals) into three major "destinations": Work, heat and storage. As the image below shows, the average number of available calories per person in the US is increasing. In general, there is more "energy in".

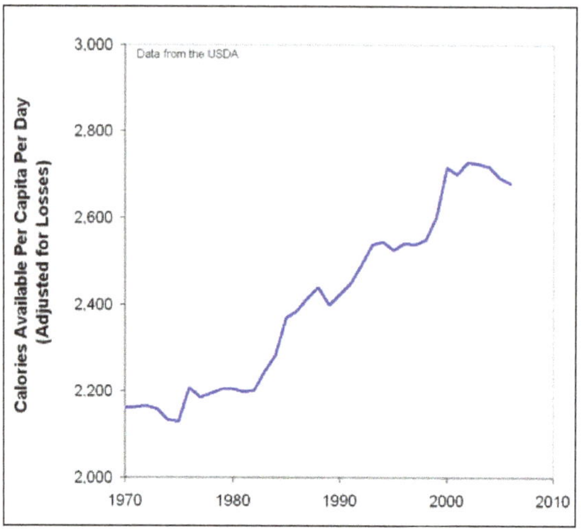

When it comes to "energy out," the body's energy needs include the amount of energy required for maintenance at rest, physical activity and movement, and for food digestion, absorption, and transport.

We can estimate our energy needs by measuring the amount of oxygen we consume. We eat, we digest, we absorb, we circulate, we store, we transfer energy, we burn the energy, and then we repeat.

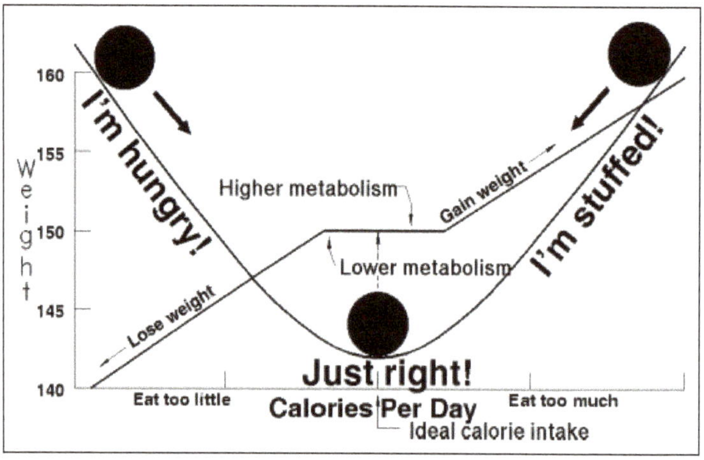

Importance of Energy Balance

There's a lot more to energy balance than a change in body weight. Energy balance also has to do with what's going on in your cells. When you're in a positive energy balance (more in than out) and when you're in a negative energy balance (more out than in), everything from your metabolism, to your hormonal balance, to your mood is impacted.

Negative Energy Balance

A severe negative energy balance can lead to a decline in metabolism, decreases in bone mass, reductions in thyroid hormones, reductions in testosterone levels, an inability to concentrate, and a reduction in physical performance.

Yet a negative energy balance does lead to weight loss. The body detects an energy "deficit" and fat reserves are called upon to make up the difference.

The body doesn't know the difference between a strict diet monitored by a physician and simply running out of food. The body just knows it isn't getting enough energy, so it will begin to slow down (or shut down) all "non-survival" functions.

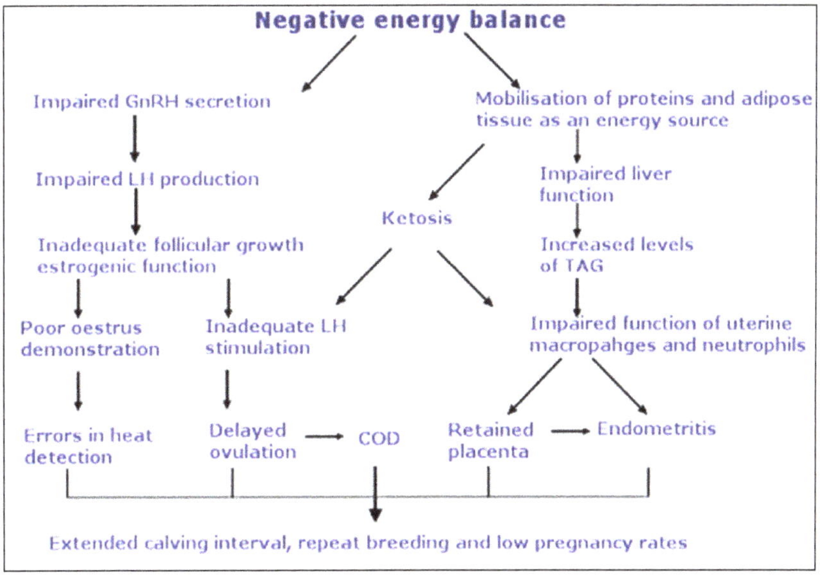

Positive Energy Balance

Overfeeding (and/or under exercising) has its own ramifications not only in terms of weight gain but in terms of health and cellular fitness. With too much overfeeding, plaques can build up in arteries, the blood pressure and cholesterol in our body can increase, we can become insulin resistant and suffer from diabetes, we can increase our risk for certain cancers, and so on.

The relationship between the amount of Calories we eat in the diet and the amount of energy we use in the body determines our body weight and overall health. The body is highly adaptable to a variety of energy intakes/outputs. It must be adaptable in order to survive. Therefore, mechanisms are in place to ensure stable energy transfer regardless of whether energy imbalances exist.

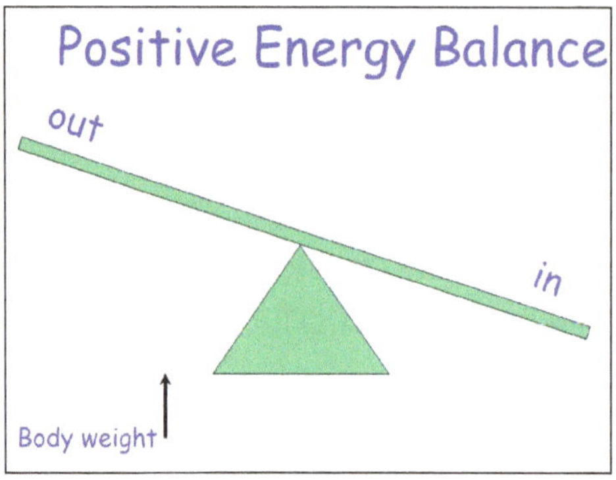

Knowing about Energy Balance

The standard "textbook" view of energy balance doesn't offer consistent explanations for body composition changes. This is because calorie restriction or over-consumption without a "metabolic intervention" (such as exercise or drugs) is likely to produce equal losses in lean mass and fat mass with restriction or equal gains in lean mass and fat mass with overfeeding.

People will likely end up as smaller or larger versions of the same shape. They'll lose muscle along with fat. Both sides of the energy balance equation are complex and the interrelationships determine body composition and health outcomes.

Gone are the days of eating a 1500 calorie meal from McDonald's and then "exercising" it off. Overall lifestyle habits help to properly control energy balance, and when properly controlled, excessive swings in either direction (positive or negative) are prevented and the body can either lose fat or gain lean mass in a healthy way.

Factors that Affect Energy In

- Calorie intake.
- Energy digested and absorbed (90-99%).

Factors that Affect Energy Out

Work

- Physical work (exercise and activity).

Heat

- Heat produced with physical work.
- Heat produced via the thermic effect of food (TEF).
- Heat produced by resting metabolism.
- Heat produced: Adipose creation.
- Heat produced: Adipose thermoregulation.

Storage

- Efficiency of work.
- Efficiency of food metabolism.
- Energy stored in adipose tissue.

Energy balance in sport and in normal daily life can help you tip the scales in your favor. However, you may be asking what is meant by energy balance and what does that mean for you?

Energy balance is the difference between your calorie consumption from food & liquid (energy intake) and calories used during daily activity, exercise and your metabolic rate (energy expenditure). By altering these you can affect your daily balance creating a positive, level or negative balance and make the difference between gaining weight and losing weight.

Loser - How to Lose Weight

Top Tips:

- Create a calorie deficit of 500 calories per day.
- Spread your calories across the day to stimulate your metabolism.
- Choose slow digesting carbohydrates, such as whole breads and pastas.
- Consume protein with each meal/snack to maintain muscle.
- Reduce your plate size and therefore your portion size for each meal.
- Aim to consume 5 portions of fruit and vegetables across the day.

Maintainer - How to Maintain Body Weight

Top Tips:

- Balance your calorie intake with your energy expenditure.

- Spread your calorie consumption to 5 meals or snacks per day.
- Select slow digesting carbohydrates as part of your diet.
- Eat a protein rich food after training to rebuild muscle.
- Consume lean proteins within each meal/snack.
- Aim to consume 5 portions of fruit and vegetables across the day.

Gainer – How to Gain Weight

Top Tips:

- Create a calorie surplus of 500 calories per day.
- Spread your calorie consumption to 5/6 meals or snacks per day.
- Choose slow digesting carbohydrates and lean proteins for each meal/snack.
- Add healthy fats to your diet as they contribute more calories than carbohydrate or protein.
- Eat a protein rich food after training to support muscle development.
- Consume a snack containing the protein casein (e.g. milk) before bed.

NIf you need to create a positive (gainer), level (maintainer) or negative (loser) energy balance for your goal, use the following equation to work out your daily calorie requirements:

Daily Energy Requirements

Step 1

First you need to calculate your Basal Metabolic rate (BMR).

MALE - BMR = 66 + (13.7 x WEIGHT (kg)) + (5 x HEIGHT (cm)) - (6.8 x AGE).

FEMALE - BMR = 655 + (9.6 x WEIGHT (kg)) + (1.8 x HEIGHT (cm)) – (4.7 x AGE).

E.g. - 1858.8 = 66 + (13.7 x 80 kg) + (5 x 172 cm) – (6.8 x 24).

Step 2

Multiply your BMR by 1.55, the activity factor for exercising 3-5 times per week.

E.g. - 1858.8 x 1.55 = 2881 calories.

Step 3

Depending on your goal, either reduce or increase your calories by 500 calories from the activity adjusted amount.

E.g. - Weight Loser: 2881 - 500 = 2381 calories.

Weight Maintainer: 2881 calories.

Weight Gainer: 2881 + 500 = 3381 calories.

Example based on male aged 24, weighing 80 kg, measuring 172cm in height. The Harris-Benedict equation (also called the Harris-Benedict principle) is a method used to estimate an individual's basal metabolic rate (BMR) and daily calorie requirements. We are all individuals, with different requirements to achieve our goals but covering the basics of consuming a healthy diet for a and suitable energy balance will create the conditions for your body to be at its best and make your goal a success.

Caloric Balance

Caloric balance refers to the number of calories you take in compared to the number of calories you burn. The principle of caloric balance matters to your overall health and fitness, because it determines whether you maintain weight, gain weight or lose weight over time. Caloric balance doesn't take into account whether calories come from proteins, carbohydrates or fats; it involves only total calories in and total calories out.

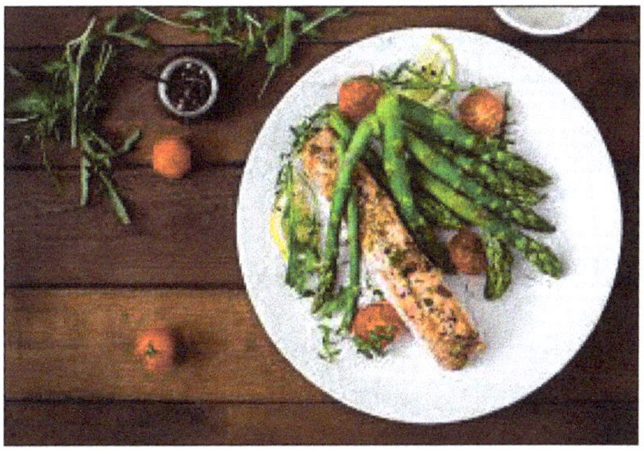

Balance

When your calorie intake and output are equal, you are in energy balance. In this state, your weight stays consistent, and you are eating enough food to support your activities of day-to-day living. The amount of calories you need to maintain this balance depends on a number of factors. For example, if you engage in high-intensity athletics, you need to consume more food than a sedentary person to account for the calories you burn during exercise. Your basal metabolic rate – the baseline caloric needs of your body's physiological functions – also impacts your caloric balance. During times of stress or fever, for instance, your basal metabolic rate increases, resulting in an increased need for calories to maintain your weight.

Excess

In caloric excess, you consume more calories than you burn on a regular basis, either intentionally or unintentionally. Intentional caloric excess can be beneficial to your health if you are underweight, ill or simply trying to pack on muscle mass. It can even be necessary, if, for example, you are pregnant or are an adolescent going through a growth spurt. On the other hand, eating more calories than you need when you don't mean to, can add unwanted body fat as excess calories are stored in your adipose tissue.

Deficit

Caloric deficit, or negative energy balance, occurs when the food calories you take in can't keep up with your body's energy needs. Deliberately keeping yourself in a caloric deficit can help you shed unwanted weight, and doing so in a gradual manner – losing no more than 1 to 2 pounds each week – helps ensure you remain healthy during your weight-loss regimen. If you find you are losing weight over time when your goal is to maintain your weight, you might be experiencing a health issue that needs your physician's attention.

Considerations

The principle of caloric balance doesn't address how nutritious your diet is. Even though you may be maintaining your weight, you might still suffer from a nutritional deficiency if your intake of proteins, carbohydrates, fats, vitamins or minerals is not well balanced. In addition, maintaining energy balance doesn't necessarily mean your body composition is ideal. Lack of lean muscle mass and an elevated level of body fat can be a sign of poor health even if your weight is stable. For overall fitness and well-being, caloric balance, nutritional status and body composition all matter.

Weight management is difficult for most individuals, as indicated by the high numbers of overweight and obese individuals in the USA and around the world. Currently, ~66 % of the US adult population is either overweight and/or obese, with ~34 % being obese. Unfortunately, the obesity epidemic is not limited to adults. Currently, 32 % of children and youth between the ages of 2 and 19 years are above the 85 % percentile for body mass index (BMI, kg/m^2) for age, which means that more young athletes will come to their sport fatter than considered desirable for optimal performance.

Although not typically obese or over fat, elite and recreational athletes can also struggle with body-weight and image issues. Depending on the sport, it is not unusual for athletes to want to lose body fat while gaining or maintaining lean tissue. While some athletes appear to be naturally lean, with weight and body size well matched for their sport, others need to change their weight and/or body composition to be competitive. If a child/youth athlete is overweight or obese, they may have a significant amount of weight to lose to be considered competitive and, thus, be pressured by themselves and others to lose weight. Youth sports programs are an optimal time to help young athletes learn to eat for health, performance, and weight management, applying the basic concepts of energy balance. Thus, there is a need for weight-management guidelines to help both elite and recreational athletes of all ages achieve an optimal body weight and composition for their sport and health.

Weight Issues in Athletes and Active Individuals

In general, most athletes and active individuals who want to lose weight fall into two categories:

- Those who are over fat or obese based on body-fat levels.
- Those who are already lean, but desire additional body fat loss. Some of these athletes fall into weight-sensitive (e.g., endurance athletes, ski jumping), weight-class (e.g., wrestling, judo), or aesthetically judged (e.g., gymnastics, figure skating) sports.

For the athlete with excess body fat, weight loss could improve sport performance and reduce the risk of chronic disease. For example, Borchers et al. found that 21 % of their Division 1 college football players (mean age, 20 years) were obese (≥25 % body fat) and had insulin resistance, while 9 % had metabolic syndrome (all obese). Thus, for these athletes, weight loss could improve performance and prevent the development of serious chronic diseases.

Conversely, many elite and recreational athletes are normal weight or have low body weights, yet they still want to lose weight to improve performance and/or to achieve a body shape for aesthetic reasons. Some of these individuals are young and still growing, which is the least desirable time to severely restrict energy intake while participating in high levels of exercise. In helping these individuals achieve their weight and sport goals, it is imperative that the risk of introducing restrictive and disordered eating behaviors is minimized, especially in those athletes participating in lean build sports. Finally, it can be difficult to manage safe weight loss in athletes who need to meet a designated weight on competition day, such as lightweight rowers, jockeys, or wrestlers. These individuals typically weight cycle, with their weight fluctuating dramatically between the competitive and off seasons. In addition, for athletes in aesthetic sports (e.g., figure skaters, synchronized swimmers, gymnasts), keeping weight low over a competitive season without injury or illness or the use of extreme weight-control methods is also a challenge. Few athletes are naturally light weight enough for these types of competitive sports, so weight loss will be required the weeks or days prior to competition.

Regardless of why the athlete needs to lose weight, working with a registered dietitian (RD) trained in sport nutrition can help the athlete identify and reach a realistic goal weight without the use of extreme diets or dangerous weight-loss practices or supplements.

Depending on the sport, the weight an athlete can maintain without dieting is typically higher than their competition weight. Thus, many athletes will restrict energy intake to achieve their competitive weight and gain weight in the off season. The ultimate goal is to identify a healthy body weight that the athlete can maintain for most of the year, while minimizing the amount of weight that needs to be lost for competition. This approach reduces the yo-yo dieting that occurs each season. For some sports, trying to maintain a low competition weight throughout the year is not possible or healthy for most athletes. The following questions can help the athlete identify whether the weight they are trying to achieve is realistic and can be maintained without constant dieting. The athlete can determine what weight works best for them during the off season and how much time they need to reach their competitive weight while remaining healthy and injury free.

- Does the goal weight minimize health issues that can increase the risk for injuries and promote good health and eating habits, while allowing for optimal sport training and performance?
- Does the goal weight take into consideration the genetic makeup and family history of body weight and shape?
- Is the goal weight appropriate for age and level of physical development, including normal reproductive function?
- Can the goal weight be maintained without constant dieting or restraining food intake, which could lead to disordered eating or an eating disorder?

Ultimately, the goal is to identify a weight that promotes good health and is 'reasonable' to achieve and maintain for most of the year, while keeping the 'diet for weight loss' periods short. An athlete who is constantly dieting or repeatedly gaining and losing weight may be trying to achieve an unrealistic body weight, which may place them at risk for disordered eating. A sport dietitian can monitor these athletes to assure they are maintaining healthy eating habits. It also requires that the medical and coaching staff know and can recognize risk factors for disordered eating when they occur and initiate early intervention.

Dynamic Energy Balance

Maintenance of body weight is an indication of being in a state of energy balance where energy intake (total kcal consumed) equals energy expenditure (total kcal expended). However, if the goal is to change energy balance, either for weight gain or weight loss, this static energy balance approach no longer applies since weight is changing. Energy balance is a dynamic process, and changing one factor on the energy intake side can also impact the energy expenditure side even without any intentional effort to alter energy expenditure. Thus, numerous factors work together to influence each side of the energy balance equation, which ultimately determines body weight. For example, total energy expenditure will be influenced by total energy intake, dietary macronutrient composition, and the energy density of the diet. These dietary factors can also alter the thermic effect of food and the type of substrates oxidized during exercise. Conversely, exercise type, duration, and intensity can alter total energy intake. For example, high-intensity exercise can blunt appetite-regulating hormones, which may ultimately lead to reduced energy intake. Other factors that can confound the assessment of energy balance in an athlete are the total amount of non-sport-related activities (e.g., walking and biking as modes of transportation, yoga, dancing, etc.) and the amount of sitting, standing, and fidgeting an athlete does. While some athletes are very active outside of training for their sport, others become quite sedentary when they are not training, which can decrease energy needs below predicted levels. Finally, assessing energy balance in a highly active athlete can also be challenging. Energy expenditure can be altered due to changes in energy efficiency and body composition with training, which may not be captured unless doubly labeled water (DLW) is used to measure energy expenditure.

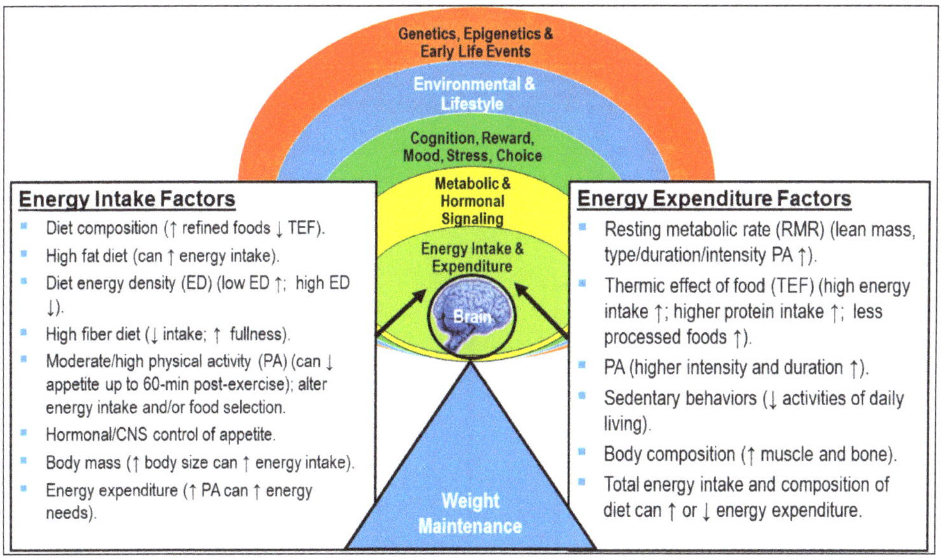

When individuals consumed a low-calorie, high-protein diet for weight loss, 1 pound (lb, 454 g) of weight lost was equal to approximately 3500 kcals. This calculation was based on examining the energy content of a pound of body fat. Many health professionals make a common mistake when explaining energy balance to athletes and active individuals. They assume that changing either side of the equation by 3500 kcal (7700 kJ) will always result in a pound of weight gained or lost, without considering all the other factors that might change as energy intake or energy expenditure is altered. Using a 75-kg man, they demonstrated how weight would change if this individual consumed an extra 100 kcal/day (~420 kJ) for 40 years. The static energy balance equation would calculate the amount of extra energy consumed to equal ~1.5 million kcal with an estimated weight gain of 417 lbs (~190 kg) over the 40-year period. Yet, intuitively, health professionals know this would not happen. The static energy balance calculation does not take into account the increase in energy expenditure that would occur as weight is gained. As weight increases, resting metabolic rate (RMR) and energy expenditure would also increase, since there is a greater energy cost in maintaining and moving a larger body. What would actually happen is that after a short period of positive energy balance, body weight would increase, resulting in an increase in energy expenditure that will eventually balance the increased energy intake. Thus, the individual would eventually achieve energy balance and become weight stable at a higher body weight, which might be a realistic weight gain of ~6 lbs. (~2.7 kg). However, to maintain this larger body size, the individual would need to continue to eat these additional kcals each day. Of course, the amount of actual weight gained will depend on a number of individual factors, extra kcal consumed, composition of the diet, body composition, type of exercise in which the individual is engaged, and overall energy expenditure.

The concept of dynamic energy balance and some of the key factors that influence each side of the energy balance equation is illustrated in Figure. How an individual responds to changes in each factor will depend on genetics, changes in regulatory hormones that control energy balance and appetite, gut health, and the food and exercise environment that can drive eating, exercise, and body composition.

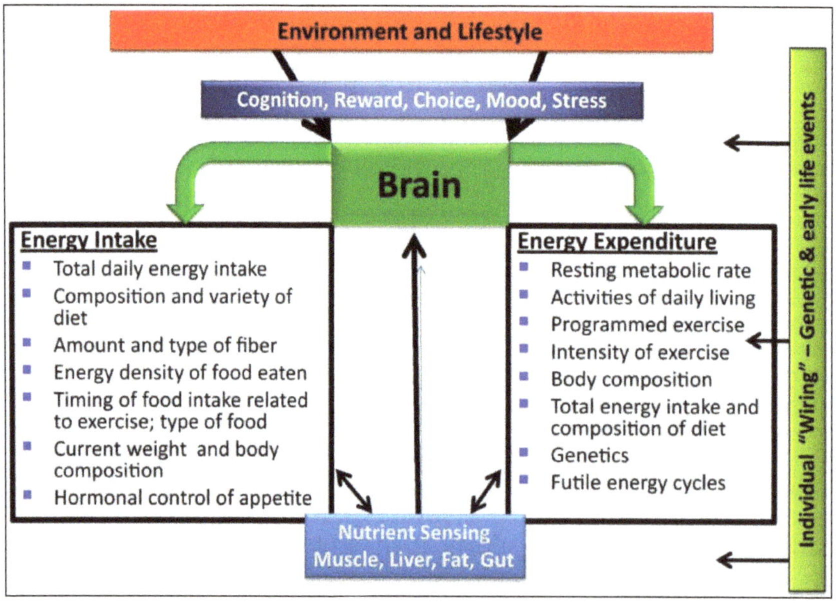

Figure: Factors regulating/influencing energy balance.

Predicting Weight Loss with Dieting

We now know that weight loss changes over time with the same level of negative energy imbalance. The energy deficit required for weight loss is less at the beginning of a diet (e.g., <3500 kcal/lb or 7700 kcal/kg), which is attributed to changes in glycogen, protein, and fluid balance. This point was demonstrated by Heymsfield et al., as they found that when overweight (BMI ~28 kg/m^2) sedentary men and women restricted energy intake by 25 %, the energy deficit required for weight loss was ~2200 kcal/lb during the first 4 weeks of the diet. As the time on the diet increased, the energy deficit required for weight loss also increased and approached Wishnofsky's 'rule' of 3500 kcal/lb by 6 months. Thus, the degree and rate at which weight loss occurs on a diet will depend on numerous factors, including the level of energy restriction, composition of the diet, total daily energy expenditure, and initial body composition.

Dietary Strategies for Weight Loss or Maintenance

What changes in diet and exercise behaviors will produce the desired body-weight and composition changes while being sustainable and manageable by the active individual? For athletes who are already very active, they will need to rely more heavily on the dietary and lifestyle strategies listed below to achieve weight loss. For athletes who are less active or not in training, increasing physical activity in addition to dietary manipulations may be necessary.

Avoid Severe Energy Restriction

It is tempting to severely restrict energy intake to get quick weight-loss results. However, this approach, combined with an intense endurance and strength-training program, can actually increase metabolic adaptations that slow weight loss and diminish the additive effects of these two factors on weight loss. Thus, this approach should be avoided. It is important to remember that with negative energy balance, lean, fit individuals can quickly lose lean tissue if energy is restricted too dramatically. For example, Pasiakos et al. placed active military personnel (BMI 25 ± 1 kg/m^2) on a 40 % energy-restricted diet for 30 days, while being fed the recommended dietary allowance (RDA) for protein (0.8 g/kg/body weight). Of the 3.3 kg lost during this time (4.2 % body weight), 58 % was lean tissue (1.9 kg). In contrast, when Redman et al. placed sedentary overweight individuals (BMI 27.8 kg/m^2) on a 25 % energy-restriction diet for 3 months, they lost 6 kg, with only 33 % coming from lean tissue (2 kg). In addition, Garthe et al. showed that slower, more reasonable weight loss in athletes (~0.7 % loss of body weight/week) helped preserve lean tissue while improving strength gains compared with more severe weight loss (1.4 % weight loss/week). Finally, severe energy restriction during times of high exercise has a number of other negative performance and health consequences for the athletes, as follows:

- Decreased sport performance effects due to decreased muscle strength, glycogen stores, concentration, coordination and training responses, and increased irritability.
- Increased negative health consequences, such as injury due to fatigue, loss of lean tissue, and poor nutrient intakes, including essential nutrients, due to limited food intake.

- Increased risk of disordered eating behaviors due to severe energy restriction.
- Increased risk of dehydration, especially if the diet is ketogenic.
- Increased emotional distress due to hunger, fatigue, and stress related to following an energy-restricted diet.

Thus, for the athlete and active individual who already have a training or fitness program, it is better to moderately restrict energy intake (e.g., 500–700 kcal/day) and take longer to reach the weight loss goal. This approach also allows the time required to adapt to new dietary habits while making sure adequate energy is available for exercise training.

Monitor Protein Intake, Quality and Timing

When energy is restricted, it is easy for protein intake to decrease at the same time that protein needs to increase with energy restriction to help preserve skeletal muscle integrity, especially in physically active individuals. In general, the protein needs of athletes are higher (1.4–1.7 g/protein/kg) than that recommended by the RDA (0.8 g/protein/kg) for non-active individuals. The amount of additional protein needed will depend on the volume and type of exercise and the level of energy restriction. For example, Mettler et al. demonstrated that increasing dietary protein during periods of severe energy restriction can help maintain lean tissue in active individuals participating in strength training while dieting. For 1 week, they placed 20 healthy resistance-trained male athletes (body fat 16–17 %, BMI 23–24 kg/m^2) on an energy-restricted diet (60 % of habitual energy intake). During this time, they were randomly assigned to either a control (1 g/protein/kg; n = 10) or treatment group (2.3 g/protein/kg; n = 10). Results showed that loss of lean mass was greater in the control group (–1.6 kg in 1 week) than in the treatment group (–0.3 kg). Thus, the higher protein intake (~35 % of energy intake) helped preserve lean tissue when energy intake was severely restricted for a short time.

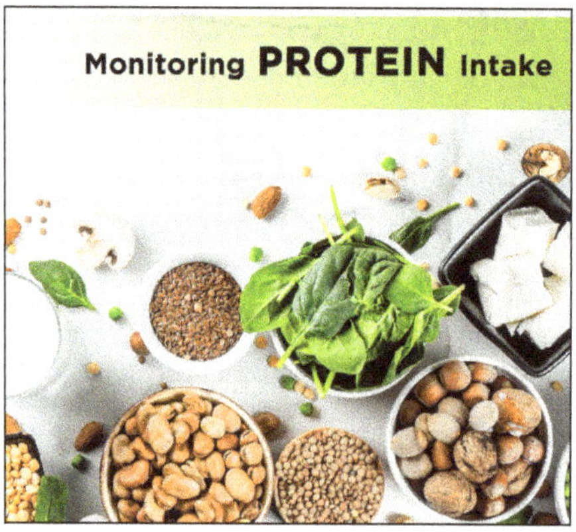

In addition to consuming more protein overall, athletes need to consume adequate high-quality protein throughout the day, but especially after exercise and at breakfast. Spreading protein intake throughout the day can benefit the athlete trying to lose weight by ensuring that adequate protein is constantly available for building, repair, and maintenance of lean tissue. Second, higher protein diets have been associated with increased satiety and reductions in energy intake. For example, Weigle et al. reported a decrease in energy intake (−441 ± 64 kcal/day) over a 12-week period in healthy sedentary individuals (BMI 26.2 ± 2.1 kg/m^2) fed an ad libitum high-protein diet (30 % energy from protein, 20 % fat, and 50 % carbohydrate) compared with an isocaloric lower protein diet (15 % of energy from protein). Although most athletes consume plenty of protein, they may not be strategic about getting this protein after exercise and spreading it out across the day. It may be more typical for the majority of the energy and protein to be consumed in a large meal at the end of the day.

Adopt a Low-Energy Dense Diet Plan

A low-ED diet is high in whole fruits, vegetables, and grains, and incorporates low-fat dairy, legumes/beans, and lean meats. Overall, the diet is lower in fat and reduces or eliminates ED beverages, especially sweetened beverages and alcohol. This high-fiber, high-water, low-fat diet means an individual can consume a greater volume of food for an overall lower energy intake and still feel satiated. The energy density of a diet or a food is determined by measuring the amount of energy (kcal) for a given amount (g) of food (kcal/day). Evidence shows that a low-ED eating plan is effective at reducing energy intake, facilitating weight loss, and preventing weight regain, and maintaining satiety in well-controlled feeding studies and in free-living conditions. For example, Bell et al. examined the effectiveness of a low-ED eating plan on total energy intake and weight loss. They found that when they fed three different levels of ED diets, the women ate a similar amount and weight of food; however, on the lowest low-ED diet condition, participants consumed 30 % less energy than the high-ED diet. Furthermore, the women did not report any differences in hunger and fullness ratings or enjoyment of the meals across test conditions. In a follow-up study, Rolls et al. examined the effect of changing portion size, energy density or a combination of the two conditions on total energy intake over 2 days. Energy density was altered by changing the portions of vegetables in entrées and by substituting low-fat foods/ingredients for full-fat foods (e.g., skim milk for whole milk). They found that energy density and portion size independently altered energy intake. When portion size was reduced by 25 %, energy intake decreased by −231 kcal/day (10 % decreases); however, reducing energy density by 25 % decreased energy intake by −575 kcal/day (24 % decrease). When both energy density and portion sizes were reduced simultaneously, energy intake decreased by 32 %. Thus, reducing portion sizes and energy density reduces energy intake; however, just reducing the energy density of the foods consumed reduces energy intake more than reducing portion sizes. Subsequent research has shown this weight loss approach also works in longer dietary interventions. Ello-Martin et al. showed that obese women counseled to consume a low-ED diet (n = 35) for 1 year lost 20 % more weight (−7.9 kg) than those counseled to reduce fat intake only (n = 36; −6.4 kg). Dietary fat intake was similarly reduced in both groups, but those in the low-ED group reported significantly lower ratings of hunger. Physical activity did not differ between the groups, with mean step counts at 8735 per day.

Currently, no published research has reported using a low-ED diet for weight loss in athletes; however, researchers have observed that female athletes with exercise-associated menstrual dysfunction who consume low-ED diets have inadequate energy intake to match energy expenditure. This research suggests that for highly active females, a low-ED diet does not provide enough energy to cover the cost of exercise and reproductive function. The satiating effect of these diets combined with the hunger-blunting effects of intense exercise may contribute to the under-eating of these athletes.

Overall, reducing the ED of the diet is more effective at lowering energy intake than is reducing portion size, without affecting hunger, fullness, or enjoyment of the food. For athletes trying to lose weight, this has important implications. It may be easier for an active individual to consume a similar amount of food and focus on changing the energy density rather than the portion sizes. This approach reduces hunger and increases adherence to the weight-loss diet plan. Finally, following a lower-ED diet could help the athlete maintain their weight loss. In summary, a key component of a low-ED eating plan is to increase the intake of foods high in water and fiber that promote satiation, while reducing both high-fat foods (i.e., potato chips, cheese, cookies) and low water and fiber foods (i.e., baked tortilla chips, pretzels). The low-ED eating plan also increases total fiber intake, which helps individuals achieve the recommended intakes.

Timing of Food Intake Around Exercise and Spreading Meals/Snacks During the Day

For the athlete, timing of food intake around exercise training and spreading food intake throughout the day will ensure that the body has the energy and nutrients needed for exercise and the building and repair of lean tissue. This approach can also prevent the athlete from becoming too hungry and consuming foods or beverages not on their diet plan. Unfortunately, when athletes attempt to lose weight, they often use unhealthy weight-loss practices such as fasting or skipping meals, severe energy restriction, and dehydration. When athletes are concerned about weight, especially female athletes, they restrict meals, especially breakfast. For example, Erdman et al. reported that nearly all (98 %) of their elite-level Canadian athletes (mean age 20.6 years, 36 % male) consumed breakfast, while Shriver et al. found that only 23 % of their Division I college-level female athletes consumed breakfast. The majority of the athletes in the Shriver et al study reported their diets to be fair/poor, ate the majority of their calories at dinner, and expressed difficulties in maintaining weight. In addition, one-third of the athletes wanted to lose weight. Thus, breakfast skipping may be a result of not making breakfast a priority or hoping that skipping a meal will help reduce overall caloric intake.

For the athlete, the breakfast or mid-morning meal is especially important because it can provide needed carbohydrates to help replenish glycogen after an overnight fast and provide fuel for exercise. For those athletes who participate in early-morning workouts, eating a light snack prior to practice and a nutritious breakfast after practice will assure that adequate nutrients are consumed, especially carbohydrate and protein. For example, Carlsohn et al. found that, for junior elite triathletes, breakfast provided 21 and 28 % of the daily carbohydrate intake during moderate- and high-intensity training weeks, respectively. Thus, skipping breakfast would mean that either total daily carbohydrate intake would be lower, potentially impacting exercise performance, or that other meals and snacks would have to provide this carbohydrate intake. Fortunately, it is easy to consume a low-ED, high-nutrient dense breakfast by including low-fat, high-quality protein (e.g., low-fat dairy or soy products, egg whites, lean meats) and high-fiber, carbohydrate-rich foods (e.g., whole grains, fruits).

Finally, refueling after exercise is still important for the athlete during weight loss. Thus, the post-exercise dietary routine needs to include fluids for rehydration, carbohydrates in the form of low-ED foods (e.g., whole fruits and vegetables, whole grains, legumes/beans) to replenish glycogen, and high-quality low-fat protein for building and repair of lean tissue. Because many athletes may not have these foods readily available after exercise, they must plan ahead and strategically use sport foods and/or health snacks to meet their energy and nutrients needs while staying within their diet plan. A sport dietitian can teach the athlete how to shop for, select, and prepare low-ED foods. Remember, the use of low-ED foods for refueling is best during training periods when there is adequate time between exercise sessions to replace muscle glycogen. During periods of competition, higher-ED foods may be required if glycogen replacement needs to occur in less than 24 h.

Reduced Consumption of Energy Dense Beverages

Consumption of ED beverages and alcohol add energy to the diet, but show reduced satiety and incomplete energy compensation. For some athletes, the elimination of ED beverages from their diet may help them achieve their weight loss goals without making any other dietary changes. For these athletes, sweetened beverages (e.g., sport drinks) should be limited to what is needed for hydration and fueling when participating in exercise and sport.

Water Balance

Osmosis is the passage of solutions across a semi-permeable membrane. Water follows the ions in an attempt to equalize the ionic concentration in the compartments on both sides of the membrane. Osmotic pressure is the pressure excreted by particles in a solution to draw water across a membrane.

Regulation of Daily Water Input

Total water output per day averages 2.5 liters. This must be balanced with water input. Our tissues produce around 300 milliliters of water per day through metabolic processes. The remainder of water output must be balanced by drinking fluids and eating solid foods. The average fluid consumption per day is 1.5 liters, and water gained from solid foods approximates 700 milliliters.

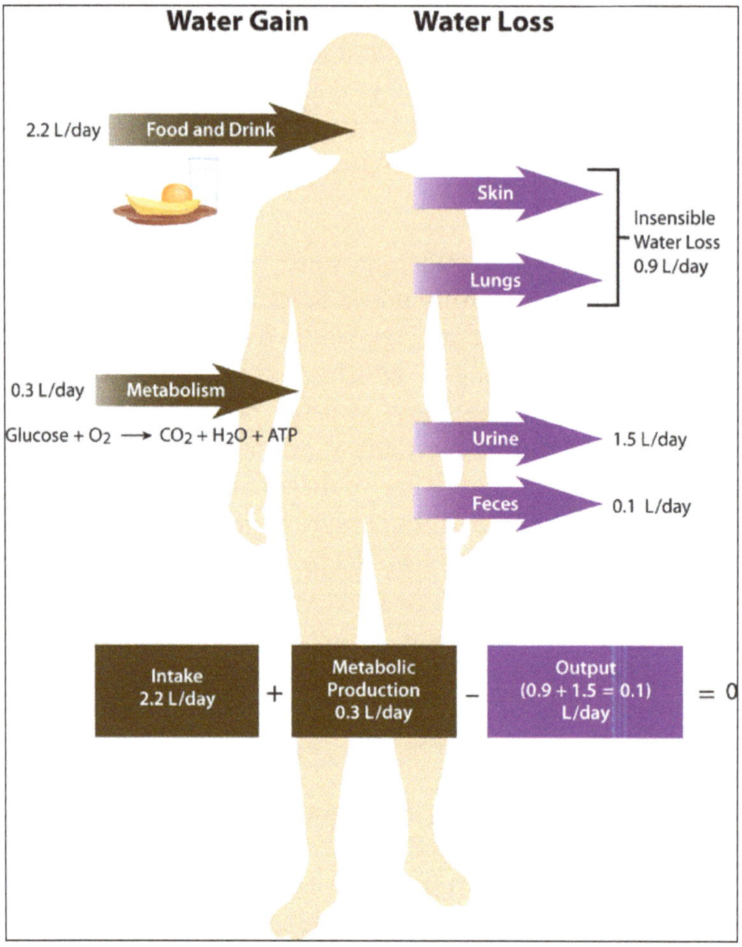

Figure: Daily Fluid Loss and Gain.

Dietary Gain of Water

The Food and Nutrition Board of the Institute of Medicine (IOM) has set the Adequate Intake (AI) for water for adult males at 3.7 liters (15.6 cups) and at 2.7 liters (11 cups) for adult females. These intakes are higher than the average intake of 2.2 liters. It is important to note that the AI for water includes water from all dietary sources; that is, water coming from food as well as beverages. People are not expected to consume 15.6 or 11 cups of pure water per day. In America, approximately 20 percent of dietary water comes from solid foods.

Table: Water Content in Foods.

Percentage	Food Item
90-99	Nonfat milk, cantaloupe, strawberries, watermelon, lettuce, cabbage, celery, spinach, squash.
80-89	Fruit juice, yogurt, apples, grapes, oranges, carrots, broccoli, pears, pineapple.
70-79	Bananas, avocados, cottage cheese, ricotta cheese, baked potato, shrimp.
60-69	Pasta, legumes, salmon, chicken breast.
50-59	Ground beef, hot dogs, steak, feta cheese.
40-49	Pizza
30-39	Cheddar cheese, bagels, bread.
20-29	Pepperoni, cake, biscuits.
10-19	Butter, margarine, raisins.
1-9	Walnuts, dry-roasted peanuts, crackers, cereals, pretzels, peanut butter.
0	Oils, sugars.

There is some debate over the amount of water required to maintain health because there is no consistent scientific evidence proving that drinking a particular amount of water improves health or reduces the risk of disease. In fact, kidney stone prevention seems to be the only premise for water consumption recommendations. You may be surprised to find out that the commonly held belief that people need to drink eight 8-ounce glasses of water per day isn't an official recommendation and isn't based on any scientific evidence! The amount of water/fluids a person should consume every day is actually variable and should be based on the climate a person lives in, as well as their age, physical activity level, and kidney function. No maximum for water intake has been set.

Thirst Mechanism

Thirst is an osmoregulatory mechanism to increase water input. The thirst mechanism is activated in response to changes in water volume in the blood but is even more sensitive to changes in blood osmolality. Blood osmolality is primarily driven by the concentration of sodium cations. The urge to drink results from a complex interplay of hormones and neuronal responses that coordinate to increase water input and contribute toward fluid balance and composition in the body. The "thirst center" is contained within the hypothalamus, a portion of the brain that lies just above the brain stem. In older people, the thirst mechanism is not as responsive and as we age there is a higher risk for dehydration. Thirst happens in the following sequence of physiological events:

- Receptor proteins in the kidney, heart, and hypothalamus detect decreased fluid volume or increased sodium concentration in the blood.

- Hormonal and neural messages are relayed to the brain's thirst center in the hypothalamus.
- The hypothalamus sends neural signals to higher sensory areas in the cortex of the brain, stimulating the conscious thought to drink.
- Fluids are consumed.
- Receptors in the mouth and stomach detect mechanical movements involved with fluid ingestion.
- Neural signals are sent to the brain and the thirst mechanism is shut off.

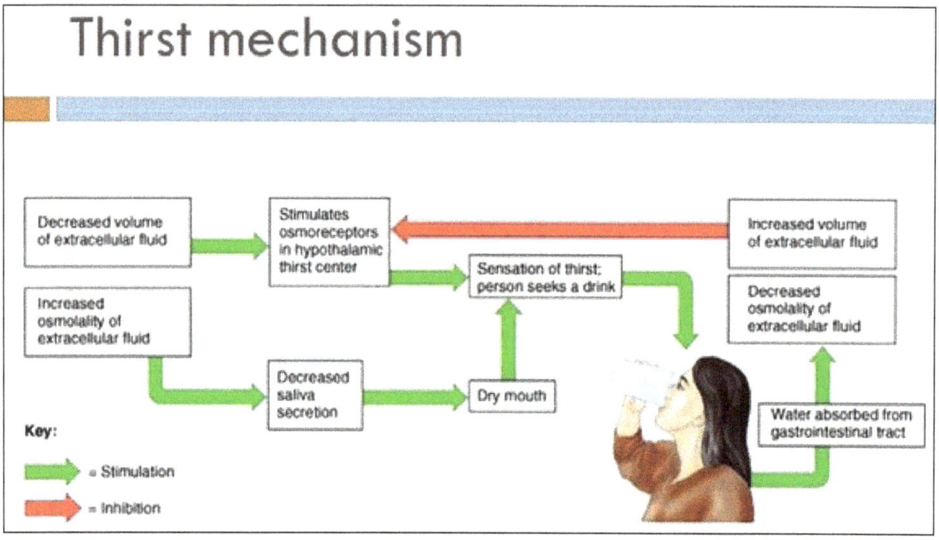

The physiological control of thirst is the backup mechanism to increase water input. Fluid intake is controlled primarily by conscious eating and drinking habits dependent on social and cultural influences. For example, you might have a habit of drinking a glass of orange juice and eating a bowl of cereal every morning before school or work. Most American adolescents have a daily habit of soft-drink consumption. Soft-drink consumption is influenced by demographics, access to soft drinks, social impacts, and personal behavior.

Regulation of Daily Water Output

Daily water output averages 2.5 liters. There are two types of outputs. The first type is insensible water loss, meaning we are unaware of it. The body loses about 400 milliliters of its daily water output through exhalation. Another 500 milliliters is lost through our skin. The second type of output is sensible water loss, meaning we are aware of it. Urine accounts for about 1,500 milliliters of water output, and feces account for roughly 100 milliliters of water output. Regulating urine output is a primary function of the kidneys, and involves communication with the brain and endocrine system.

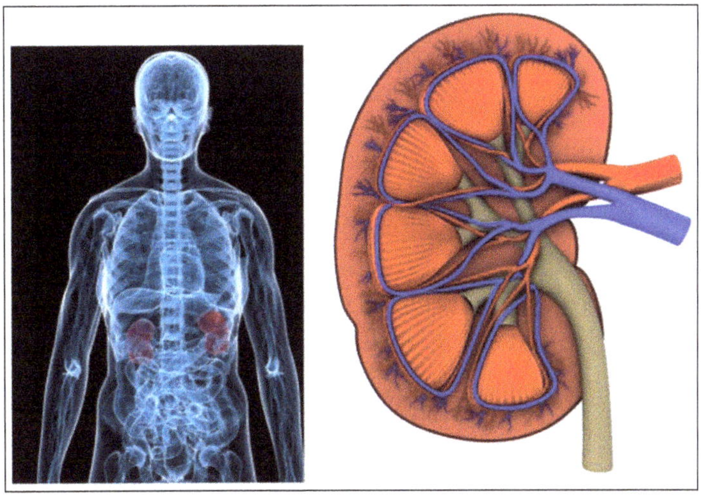

Figure: Kidneys, A primary function of the kidneys is to filter blood and remove wastes. They play a major role in fluid and electrolyte balance.

The Kidneys Detect Blood Volume

The kidneys are two bean-shaped organs, each about the size of a fist and located on either side of the spine just below the rib cage. The kidneys filter about 190 liters of blood and produce (on average) 1.5 liters of urine per day. Urine is mostly water, but it also contains electrolytes and waste products, such as urea. The amount of water filtered from the blood and excreted as urine is dependent on the amount of water in, and the electrolyte composition of, blood.

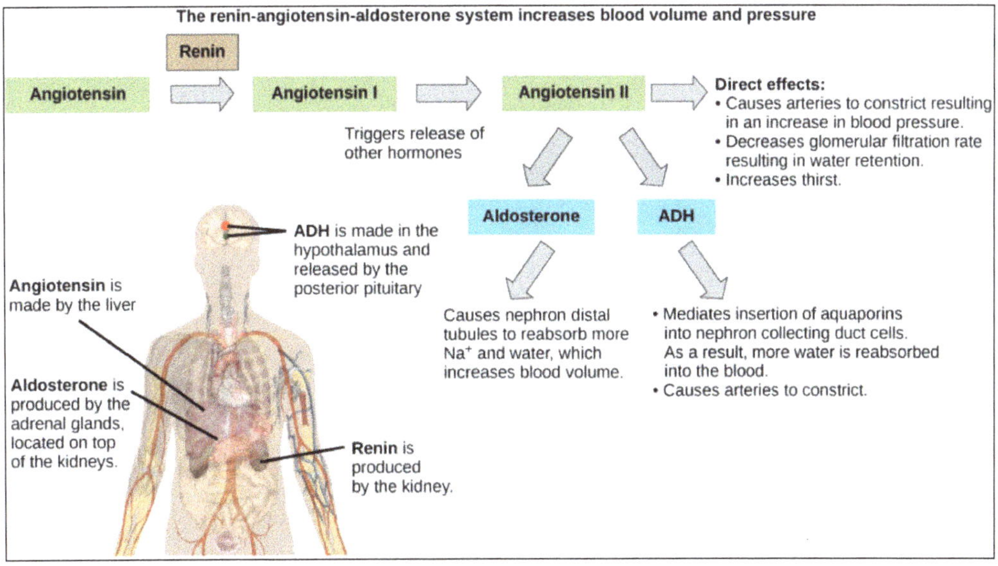

Kidneys have protein sensors that detect blood volume from the pressure, or stretch, in the blood vessels of the kidneys. When blood volume is low, kidney cells detect decreased pressure and secrete the enzyme, renin. Renin travels in the blood and cleaves another protein into the active hormone, angiotensin. Angiotensin targets three different organs (the adrenal glands, the hypothalamus, and the muscle tissue surrounding the arteries) to rapidly restore blood volume and, consequently, pressure.

- First, angiotensin travels to the outer perimeter of the adrenal glands and stimulates the release of the hormone aldosterone. Aldosterone travels back to the kidneys and stimulates the sodium-potassium pump. As a result of the pump's work, the blood reabsorbs the sodium from the liquid that has already been filtered by the kidneys. Water follows sodium into the blood by osmosis, resulting in less water in the urine and restored fluid balance and composition of blood.
- Next, angiotensin travels to the hypothalamus where it stimulates the thirst mechanism and the release of antidiuretic hormone. Antidiuretic hormone travels back to the kidneys where it increases sodium and water reabsorption.
- Lastly, angiotensin targets smooth muscle tissue surrounding arteries, causing them to contract (narrow) the blood vessels, which assists in elevating blood pressure.

The Hypothalamus Detects Blood Osmolality

Osmoreceptors (specialized protein receptors) in the hypothalamus detect sodium concentration in the blood. In response to a high sodium level, the hypothalamus activates the thirst mechanism and concurrently stimulates the release of antidiuretic hormone. Thus, it is not only kidneys that stimulate antidiuretic- hormone release, but also the hypothalamus. This dual control of antidiuretic hormone release allows for the body to respond to both decreased blood volume and increased blood osmolality.

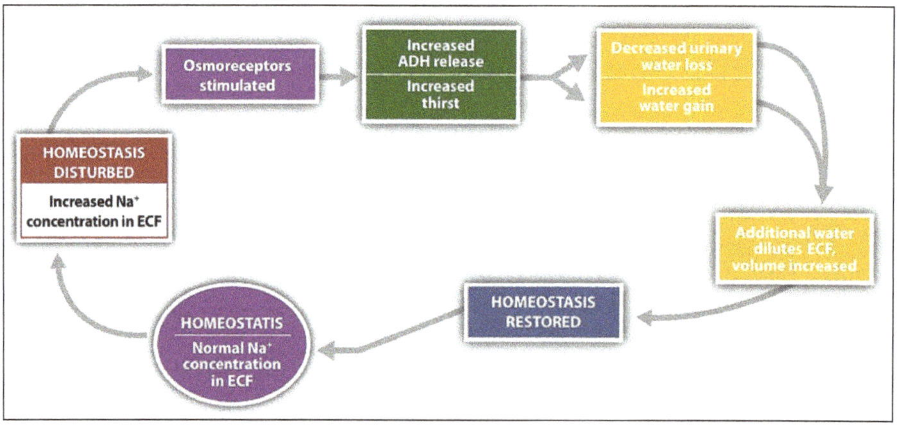

Figure: Sodium and fluid balance are intertwined.

The Adrenal Glands Detect Blood Osmolality

Cells in the adrenal glands sense when sodium levels are low, and when potassium levels are high, in the blood. In response to either stimulus, they release aldosterone.

Therefore, aldosterone is released in response to angiotensin stimulation and is also controlled by blood electrolyte concentrations. In either case, aldosterone communicates the same message, which is to increase sodium reabsorption and consequently water reabsorption. In exchange, potassium is excreted.

The mechanisms involved in regulating water input and output are intertwined with those controlling electrolyte balances. In a healthy individual, this multilevel coordinated control of fluid and electrolyte levels in the body ensures homeostasis. However, in a person with heart failure, the crosstalk between organs can have dire consequences. Heart failure results in a decrease in blood output from the heart, which lowers blood pressure. In response to the lower blood pressure, the kidneys release renin leading to the release of antidiuretic hormone. Antidiuretic hormone acts on the kidneys and increases water reabsorption, thereby increasing blood volume and pressure. This makes the heart work harder and exacerbates the heart condition. To block this response, people with heart failure are treated with drugs that block the kidneys' compensatory response. Diuretics are drugs that act either by inhibiting the actions of antidiuretic hormone or by promoting sodium excretion in the urine. This increases water output and blood pressure is reduced. Diuretics, along with other drugs, are useful in treating heart failure and in decreasing blood pressure in people with hypertension.

Fluids in Sports

Water is essential to maintain blood volume, regulate body temperature and allow muscle contractions to take place. During exercise, the main way the body maintains optimal body temperature is by sweating. Heat is removed from the body when beads of sweat on the skin evaporate, resulting in a loss of body fluid. Sweat production, and therefore fluid loss, increases with a rise in ambient temperature and humidity, as well as with an increase in exercise intensity.

Drinking fluid during exercise is necessary to replace fluids lost in sweat. This action will reduce the risk of heat stress, maintain normal muscle function, and prevent performance decreases due to dehydration. In most cases during exercise, the rates of sweat loss are higher than the rate you can drink, so most athletes get into fluid deficit. Therefore, fluid guidelines promote drinking more fluid to reduce the deficit and potential performance detriments associated with dehydration. However, it is also important to acknowledge that it is possible to over-drink during exercise. This highlights the importance of getting to know your sweat rate and knowing how much you should be drinking.

Dehydration and Performance

As dehydration increases, there is a gradual reduction in physical and mental performance. There is an increase in heart rate and body temperature, and an increased perception of how hard the exercise feels, especially when exercising in the heat. Studies show that loss of fluid equal to 2% of body mass is sufficient to cause a detectable decrease in performance (that's a 1.4 kg loss in a 70 kg athlete).Dehydration of greater than 2% loss of body weight increases the risk of nausea, vomiting, diarrhoea, and other gastro-intestinal problems during exercise.

Dehydration reduces the rate of fluid absorption from the intestines, making it more difficult to reverse the fluid deficit. You may end up feeling bloated and sick if you delay fluid replacement. It is impossible to 'train' or 'toughen' your body to handle dehydration.

Drinking Too Much

Drinking more fluid than is comfortable, in any conditions, has the potential to interfere with your performance. In cool weather or when the exercise pace is gentle, the rate of sweat loss may be quite low. It is unnecessary and potentially dangerous to drink at rates that are far greater than sweat losses. Such over-hydration during exercise can cause a dilution of blood sodium levels (hyponatraemia). Symptoms include headaches, disorientation, coma, and in severe cases, death. It is important to note though that this is relatively rare and dehydration is a much more common issue.

Estimating your Fluid Losses

Knowing your sweat rate can give you an indication of how much you should be drinking during exercise. Sports dietitians routinely measure an athlete's sweat rate during training and competition in a range of environmental conditions, to provide them with the information required to design an individual fluid plan. Follow these easy steps to measure your fluid losses:

- Weigh yourself in minimal clothing, as close to the start of exercise as possible. Ideally you should empty your bladder before weighing.
- Commence exercise session.
- Weigh yourself at the end of your session, in minimal clothing again, ensuring you towel off any excess sweat from your body.
- Your weight change during exercise reflects your total fluid loss; i.e. the difference between your sweat losses and fluid intake.
- Remember that weight loss during exercise is primarily water loss (not fat loss), and needs to be replaced soon after finishing exercise.
- Other minor losses come from breathing, spitting, vomiting and other insignificant sources. Sweat losses can be monitored to give you an idea of how much fluid to replace during training sessions and competition.

Intake of Fluid

Drinking fluid during exercise helps to prevent a drop in performance caused by dehydration, and fluid after exercise will re-hydrate you. The amount of fluid and the timing of drinks depend on the individual and the sport. Here are some tips:

- Always start exercise well hydrated; this will lower the risk of becoming dehydrated during sport. There is minimal performance benefit to being over-hydrated as drinking excessive amounts of fluid before exercise causes increased urination and feeling bloated.
- Develop a plan for drinking during exercise based on your own sweat rates.
- Immediately after exercise, monitor your weight change to estimate your final fluid deficit. During recovery, you will continue to lose fluids through sweating and urine losses, so plan to replace 125-150% of this fluid deficit over the next 2-6 hours. For example, if you lost 1 kg (1000mL), you will need to drink 1250-1500mL to fully re-hydrate. Drink fluids with your recovery snacks and the following meal to achieve this goal.
- Different sports pose different challenges and opportunities for optimal hydration. For team and racquet sports there are formal breaks between play, with substitutions and time-outs, all offering an opportunity to drink. Some individual sports require you to drink on the move. Be smart and practice strategies to get maximum benefit from fluid intake with minimal fuss and discomfort. Try special squeeze bottles, or hands free drink pouches if practical.
- Thirst is not an effective indicator of hydration status while exercising. There is usually a significant fluid loss before you feel thirsty. When drinking, your thirst will be satisfied well before these losses have been fully replaced. What is the best fluid to drink? As there are many drink options available, you now need to think about which is best for you. Plain water alone is an effective drink for fluid replacement, especially in low intensity and short duration sports. However, if carbohydrate and electrolytes are added to water, as in a sports drink, performance can be enhanced, especially in high intensity and endurance sports.
- If a drink tastes good, athletes will consume more of it, which may assist in meeting fluid targets during competition or rehydrating more effectively. Carbohydrate in fluid provides a muscle energy source as well as enhancing flavour. This can be one advantage of a sports drink over plain water. Electrolytes such as sodium are lost in sweat and need to be replaced during and after prolonged exercise. Sodium in fluid improves fluid intake as it stimulates the thirst mechanism, promotes both carbohydrate and water uptake in the intestines, and reduces the volume of urine produced post-exercise. Of course, salt can be consumed in foods that are eaten at the same time as post-exercise fluids.

Caffeine

There are growing numbers of drinks on the market that contain a number of ingredients including caffeine. Caffeine is no longer banned by the World Anti-Doping Agency. The consumption of small to moderate doses of caffeine (75 - 200 mg) can help to sustain exercise performance, reduce the perception of effort, and is unlikely to alter hydration status during exercise. However, the use of caffeine amongst athletes is often ad hoc and they may be unaware of the potential detrimental side effects associated with its use.

Alcohol

Alcohol is not a suitable fluid to choose immediately after exercise, as it will impair vital recovery processes, and may also impair the athlete's ability to rehydrate effectively. If you choose to drink alcohol after exercise, look after your recovery needs first (i.e. replacing fluids, carbohydrate stores and consuming some protein to assist with muscle repair) and then enjoy an alcoholic beverage in sensible amounts.

Hydration

Hydration is the process of maintaining the right volume of water and electrolytes in your body. It's all about striking the balance between fluids in and fluids out. Your body relies on water and electrolytes for a number of reasons. Water plays a key role in maintaining body temperature, assisting with digestion and lubricating your tissues and joints. Electrolytes help your body to retain fluid and are essential for nerve and muscle function. When you're an active participant in sport, you rely on your muscles and joints to perform well. Keeping them well hydrated is pretty important.

Dehydration occurs when too much fluid – which includes water and electrolytes – is lost through sweat, saliva, urine and other bodily processes. In fact, you only have to lose as little as 2% of your body weight for signs of dehydration to show.

These signs can include a dry mouth, increased thirst, muscle cramping, fatigue and a lack of concentration. You may also have decreased urine output, which is a lot darker in colour than usual.

When you're exercising, dehydration can cause cramps, increased heart rate, fatigue, impaired concentration and nausea. Not ideal when you're trying to do your best gym session or play your best game of sport.

Staying Hydrated

To avoid dehydration, you need to make sure you're getting enough fluids and electrolytes before, during and after exercise. Hydralyte Sports contains the right balance of essential electrolytes and minerals your body needs – particularly if sweating has depleted your electrolyte levels.

Rapid and effective rehydration depends on activation of the sodium glucose co-transport pump within the intestinal lumen. Hydralyte Sports contains the correct balance of glucose and sodium to activate this pump, enabling the rapid influx of sodium, glucose, water (by osmosis) and other electrolytes.

Maintaining euhydration, the state of preserving body water within its optimal homeostatic range, is essential to sustain life. Water contributes 50–70% of total body mass and is compartmentalized within both intracellular (65%) and extracellular (35%) spaces. Euhydration is typically maintained over the course of day-to-day life via behavioral and biological controls. However, exercise can cause an acute disruption to fluid balance, challenging the athlete's goal of optimal performance and safety during exercise, especially in hot environmental conditions. The process of incurring a fluid deficit is known as dehydration, while the outcome is defined as hypohydration. The loss of body water during exercise exacerbates physiological and perceptual strain and it is well established that these changes can impair endurance performance, particularly in hot environments and may increase the risk of exertional heat illness.

While the sensation of thirst, a centrally mediated response to body water deficits, is useful in dictating the need for fluid intake during daily life, thirst is relatively insensitive in acutely tracking hydration status during exercise. Maintaining an optimal state of hydration during exercise becomes more complicated depending on the sport, type of activity and availability of fluid. Optimal hydration is dependent on many factors but can generally be defined during exercise as avoiding losses greater than 2–3% of body mass while also avoiding over hydration. Furthermore, during exercise, it is not uncommon for individuals to involuntarily dehydrate, in which they consume less fluid than their fluid needs. Excessive fluid intake can also be problematic, with hyponatremia developing in severe cases of over hydration. Inappropriate management of fluid intake resulting in hypohydration, or hyperhydration, can be detrimental for performance and in some circumstances, increases health risk.

Current consensus recommends that good hydration practices include:

- Beginning exercise in a state of euhydration.
- Preventing excessive hypohydration during exercise.
- Replacing remaining losses following exercise prior to the next exercise bout.

These practices attenuate the adverse effects of acute dehydration on physical activity and health. However, it is acknowledged that fluid needs are individualistic and rely on factors such as personal sweat rate, exercise mode, exercise intensity, environmental conditions and exercise duration. Furthermore, characteristics and rules unique to each sport environment in which it is played, event uniform and equipment, and the availability of fluid during both training and competition may greatly influence the ability to optimize hydration during activity.

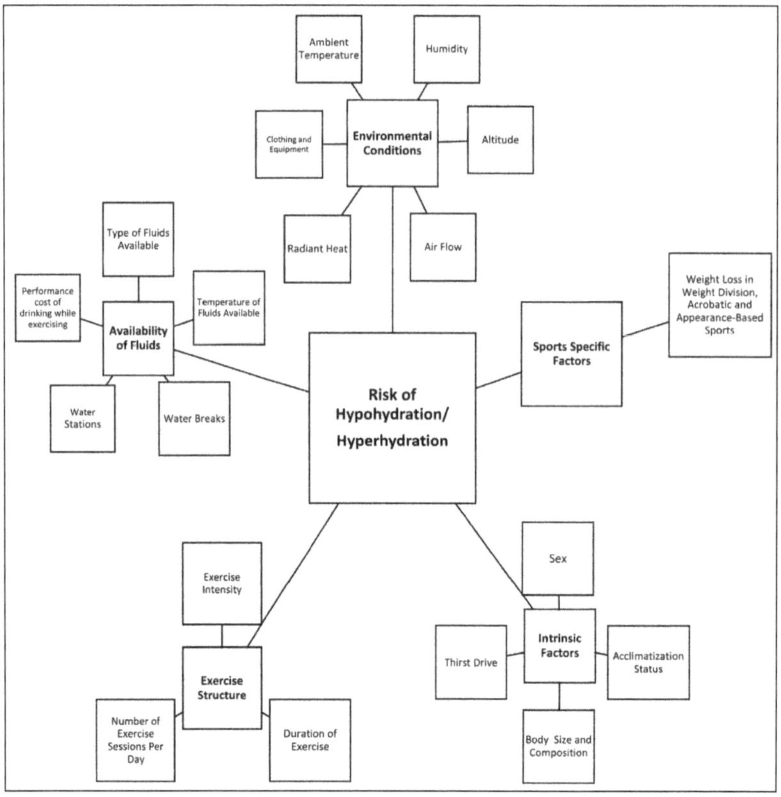

Figure: Factors that contribute to the risk of hypohydration or hyperhydration during exercise.

Hydration Assessment

Hydration assessment can be utilized to indicate one's current hydration state, but if taken serially, it can also be used to track changes in hydration and indicate fluid needs (i.e., during a bout of physical activity). While various methods of hydration assessment exist, there is no single method that can serve as a criterion measure to assess hydration status in all settings (i.e., day-to-day life and exercise, etc.). Plasma osmolality, changes in plasma volume, and the volume, osmolality and specific gravity of urine are the most commonly published metrics to assess changes in hydration status in clinical settings. The use of these measures in field applications is often impractical, due to the methods or equipment needed to acquire the measure (e.g., a needle stick to draw blood or providing a urine sample) as well as the sensitivity of the measure.

In field applications, the careful assessment of changes in body mass over a bout of physical activity provides a reasonably accurate assessment of body water deficits incurred during the session, since sweat loss and fluid intake during the session underpin the major changes in body mass and body water content. This is true for most sporting activities conducted over a duration of <2–3 h; however, during very prolonged and strenuous exercise (e.g., ultra-endurance races), other factors that cause mass changes, metabolic water production and the liberation of stored water become numerically important and undermine the utility of this assessment. A comparison of body mass pre- and post-exercise will help guide the athlete in understanding whether their hydration strategy during activity was effective in achieving acceptable fluid balance as well as knowing the volume of fluids that are needed following exercise to return to baseline hydration levels prior to the next exercise session. The methodology for assessing sweat losses is to assess the athlete's body mass before and after exercise with care to avoid or account for substantial amounts of fluid trapped in hair and clothes. Accounting for any fluid consumed or urine excreted, the difference between the masses can be used to calculate the amount of sweat lost as well as the residual fluid deficit that should be addressed in post-exercise recovery plans.

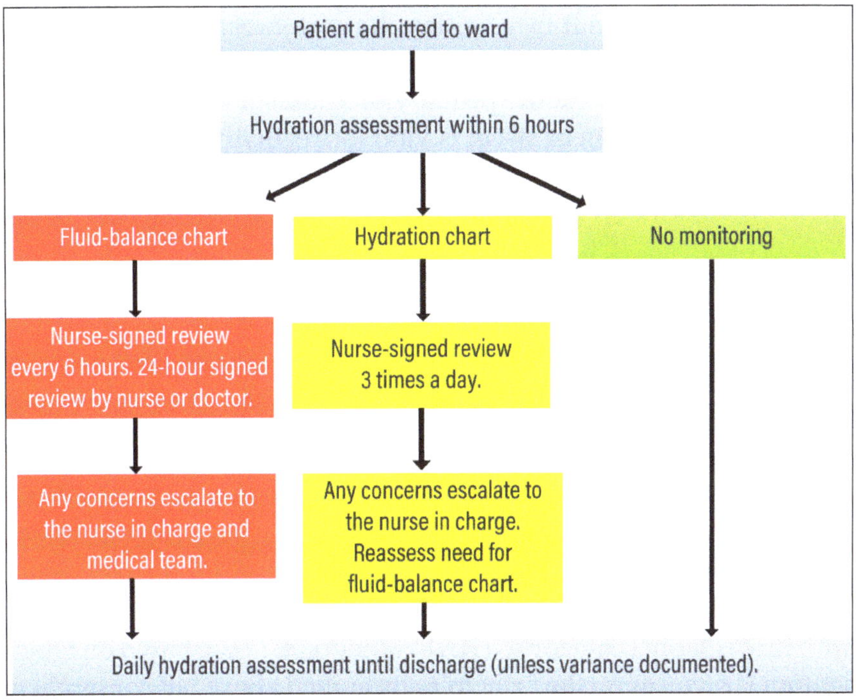

A useful paradigm for tracking daily changes in hydration status in sporting situations is to consider a combination of assessments to track daily changes. The monitoring of daily changes in body mass, coupled with urine color and thirst sensation status provides adequate sensitivity for most athletic situations. Cheuvront and Kenefick established useful criteria for these variables as body mass changes greater than 1.1%, a conscious desire for water (thirst), and dark-colored urine (>5 a.u. on an 8-a.u. scale) indicating varying degrees of fluid inadequacy. Two of these factors combined suggest daily fluid intake is likely inadequate, while all three factors indicate that daily fluid intake is very likely inadequate. It should be noted that this assessment technique is based on first morning values and requires baseline body mass values to provide the most useful information to athletes.

Practical Solutions:

- Carefully monitor acute changes in body mass over an exercise bout to determine sweat rate, adequacy of fluid replacement and fluid needs for recovery for that session. Consider how well this can be used to evaluate general hydration strategies in similar situations.
- Use changes in body mass, urine color and thirst upon awakening to track daily changes in hydration status.

Exercise Structure

Body fluid loss during sport or exercise largely results from sweating. Net fluid balance is modulated to a certain extent by drinking. Rate of sweating is primarily a function of metabolic heat production, but can be modified by environment, clothing, acclimatization and hydration status. As the primary mechanism of heat dissipation in many environments, the evaporation of sweat is vital for regulating body temperature, even during exercise in temperate weather. However, this heat dissipation is accompanied by typical fluid losses of ~0.5–1.9 L/h.

Exercise intensity is the main factor that determines metabolic heat production, meaning that the rate of fluid losses from sweat for a given exercise session can be partially explained by the intensity of the exercise. Total fluid losses are a result of the sweat rate of a given exercise intensity and the total duration of that activity. In most circumstances there is an inverse relationship between the exercise intensity of a session and the duration of that session. However, given the wide variability in individual sweat rates, the unique interplay between intensity, duration and sweat rate must be considered in unison. For example, a runner with a 2 L/h sweat rate who completes a marathon in 2 h will accumulate the same fluid losses as a runner with a 1 L/h sweat rate that completes the race in 4 h. In given tables we define exercise intensity of a range of sporting activities into three distinct categories (High, Moderate, Low), based on typical practice and competition structures on the principles described above but comprehensive plans should consider individual athletes.

Table: Team Sport Factors That Influence Hypohydration.

Sport	Availability of Fluid		Environment		Intensity		Hypohydration Risk	
	Training	Competition	Training	Competition	Training	Competition	Training	Competition
Basketball	High	High	Low	Low	Mod	Mod	Low	Low
Ice Hockey	High	High	Low	Low	Mod	High	Mod	Mod
Football	High	High	Mod	Mod	Mod	High	Mod	Mod
Baseball	High	High	Mod	Mod	Low	Low	Low	Low

Softball	High	High	Mod	Low	Low	Low	Low	Low
Volleyball	High	High	Low	Low	Low	Low	Low	Low
Soccer	High	Low	Mod	Mod	Mod	High	Mod	High
Lacrosse	High	High	Mod	Mod	Mod	Mod	Mod	Mod
Rugby	High	Low	Mod	Mod	Mod	High	Mod	High

Availability of Fluid: High, the dynamics of the sport allow for multiple opportunities to consume fluid; Moderate (Mod), Fluid is only available during breaks in training, competition, or carried by the athlete; Low, Fluid is limited or not available due to time restrictions, rules or dynamics of the sport, and ability to carry. Environment: High, environmental conditions that are of great risk for hypohydration; Mod, the environment is variable ranging from cool to hot conditions that may pose risk for hypohydration; Low, the environmental conditions are not a threat to hypohydration. Intensity: High, exercise intensity in the sport is increased and likely to result in large sweat losses and hypohydration; Mod, exercise intensity in the sport varies from moderate to high and may result in large sweat losses and hypohydration; Low, exercise intensity in the sport is low and less likely to result in large sweat losses and hypohydration. Hypohydration Risk: High, the risk for hypohydration in the sport is high based on reported sweat losses, the availability of fluid, environmental conditions, and the intensity of exercise; Mod, the risk for hypohydration in the sport is moderate based on reported sweat losses, the availability of fluid, environmental conditions, and the intensity of exercise; Low, the risk for hypohydration in the sport is low based on reported sweat losses, the availability of fluid, environmental conditions, and the intensity of exercise.

Table: Individual Sport factors that influence Hypohydration.

Sport	Availability of Fluid		Environment		Intensity		Hypohydration Risk	
	Training	Competition	Training	Competition	Training	Competition	Training	Competition
Tennis	High	Mod	Mod	Mod	High	High	Mod	Mod
Wrestling	High	High	Mod	Mod	High	High	High	Mod
Gymnastics	High	High	Low	Low	Mod	Low	Low	Low
Running(<1h)	Low	High	Mod	Mod	High	High	Low	Low
Running (1-2h)	Low	High	Mod	Mod	Mod	Mod	Mod	Mod
Running (>2h)	Low	High	Mod	Mod	Low	Mod	Mod	Mod
Cycling (<1h)	High	High	Mod	Mod	High	High	Low	Low
Cycling (>2h)	Mod	Mod	Mod	Mod	Mod	Mod	Low	High
Swimming	High	High		High	High	High	Low	Low
Triathlon (<2 h)								
Swim	Low	Low	Low	Low	Mod	Mod	Low	Low
Bike	Mod	High	Mod	Mod	Mod	Mod	Low	Low
Run	Low	High	Mod	Mod	Mod	Mod	Low	Low
Triathlon (2–5 h)								

Swim	Low	Low	Low	Low	Mod	Mod	Low	Low
Bike	Mod	High	Mod	Mod	Mod	Mod	Low	Low
Run	Low	High	Mod	Mod	Mod	Mod	Mod	Mod
Triathlon 95-9h)								
Swim	Low	Low	Low	Low	Mod	Mod	Low	Low
Bike	Mod	High	Mod	Mod	Mod	Mod	Mod	Mod
Run	Low	High	Mod	Mod	Mod	Mod	Mod	Mod
Triathlon (>9h)								
Swim	Low	Low	Low	Low	Mod	Mod	Low	Low
Bike	Mod	High	Mod	Mod	Mod	Mod	Mod	Mod
Run	Low	High	Mod	Mod	Mod	Mod	Mod	Mod

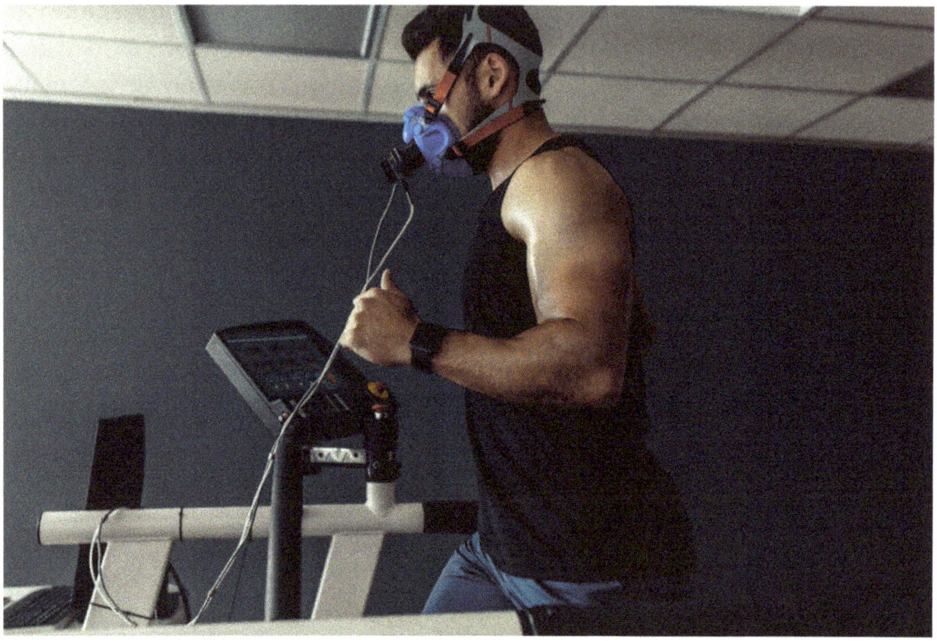

For sports like cycling and running, the influence of exercise intensity and duration on fluid needs is very easy to determine given the consistent nature of exercise. Figure below demonstrates the relationship between duration and target fluid replacement for steady-state exercise. However, as shown in Table some of the most common sports involve supramaximal exercise in short bursts with longer breaks. In this case, individuals should regard an overall average of exercise intensity rather than the maximal effort during the exercise bout when determining optimal fluid balance.

The 70 kg athlete in the example would need to drink a volume of fluid equal to 2.6 ± 0.7 L to prevent >2 ± 1% dehydration when losing 4 L of body water, such as during a marathon (42.1 km). During shorter distances such as 5 or 10 km when fluid losses are unlikely to reach or exceed 2% dehydration, the same athlete would not need to ingest fluids during competition as fluid losses accumulate to <2% dehydration.

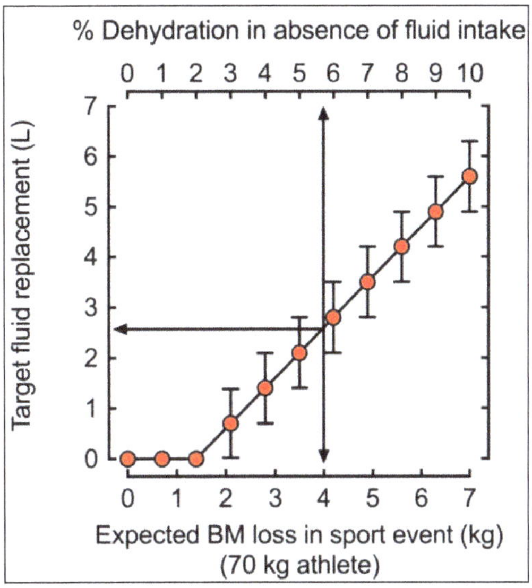

Figure: Target fluid replacement estimates to prevent >2 ± 1 % body mass (BM) loss as water (i.e., dehydration).

It should also be noted that exercise intensity influences gastric emptying rate. Individuals striving to closely match sweat losses with fluid consumption can be challenged by maximal gastric emptying rates. However, when vigorous exercise is conducted (>70% VO_{2max}), gastric emptying decreases predictably, most likely based on decreased splanchnic perfusion. Practical Solutions:

- Increased fluid intake is necessary with prolonged or intense exercise due to increased sweat production.
- During vigorous exercise (>70% VO_{2max}) understand that gastric emptying may limit fluid absorption. Athletes can train their gut to improve gastrointestinal comfort or adopt strategies to increase fluid intake before and after exercise.

Environment

At fixed exercise intensity, the ambient environment further modulates sweat rate. The magnitude of evaporative, radiant, convective and conductive heat exchange between the body and the environment is a function of the gradients between the environment and the skin which provides the main physiological interface for heat exchange. A number of factors contribute to sweat rate including ambient and radiant temperature, humidity, clothing, and air velocity, all of which differ depending on the sport or activity. Therefore, individuals exercising in hot-humid environments with direct sunlight and minimal airflow will produce near maximal sweat rates and be at the greatest risk of hypohydration. Wet-bulb globe thermometry (WBGT) accounts for these environmental factors and can help inform fluid replacement decision.

All clothing provides insulation and presents a barrier to heat loss, resulting in increased sweat rates to provide similar cooling to an unclothed situation. Thus, sports/activities with specific clothing requirements, such as American football, are at greater risk of body fluid loss compared to similar activities in which clothing is minimal. Synthetic wicking materials can increase sweat fluid losses compared to cotton garments, potentially decreasing the thermal load but increasing the risk of dehydration. When the effects of hot, humid environmental conditions are combined with clothing and equipment, individuals can achieve near maximal sweat rates which can create a significant fluid deficit rapidly.

Other Environmental Considerations

Exercising in the cold or at high altitudes merits special considerations when determining the fluid needs of athletes. Athletes must also be vigilant and mindful of their fluid needs during exercise in the cold. Exercise in the cold can still produce copious sweating, especially when heavy clothing is worn, while also diminishing thirst sensitivity and reducing *ad libitum* fluid consumption, thus potentially leading to impaired fluid replacement and hypohydration. If possible, athletes should know their individual fluid replacement needs, based upon sweat rate measurement, during exercise in hot and cold environments to ensure they can develop a plan for competing while optimally hydrated.

Athletes unaccustomed to exercising in higher altitudes may require additional fluids. Very high altitude (4900–7600 m) exposure tends to increase water and electrolyte losses, decrease plasma volume and total body water content. In both cold air and high altitudes, respiratory water losses may increase and require additional fluid consumption due to low air water vapor pressures. Therefore, athletes should acclimate to altitude over several days and maintain euhydration prior to competition to ensure optimal athletic performance.

Given tables summarizes typical environmental conditions found among a range of sports into three distinct categories, and how these conditions contribute to the considerations around an individualized fluid plan. Of course, there are large regional differences in environmental conditions experienced for sports at the same time of year. Local measurements utilizing WBGT allow for the greatest characterization of the environmental demands placed on athletes during exercise in the heat. Practical Solutions:

- Measure local environmental conditions to determine the risk of high sweat rates resulting in large fluid losses.
- Increase fluid-replacement during exercise in hot and humid environments to account for increased sweat losses.

- Account for clothing or equipment requirements when evaluating fluid needs.
- Modify fluid intake when exercising in cold or altitude according to an estimation of fluid losses noting that thirst may be less reliable as a guide to dehydration under these conditions.

Fluid Availability

Fluid availability refers to the factors that dictate an athlete's ability to replace fluid losses during activity. In many instances, the characteristics of the sport have a strong influence on the ability to drink during competition and in many scenarios prevent an athlete from "drinking to thirst". Meanwhile, training activities are often easily modified to allow for some degree of fluid replacement. In many instances, water-breaks during training can be determined on the basis of work-to-rest ratios set by environmental conditions with free access to fluid throughout the break. Characteristics such as flavor and temperature affect the palatability of fluids and may increase voluntary intake when they are matched to the cultural preferences of the athletes and the prevailing conditions (e.g., cool drinks in a warm environment).

In endurance sports which provide competitors with feed zones/water stations (e.g., running events), the number of water stations on a course and the frequency with which a competitor reaches them can influence drinking behavior. The International Association of Athletics Federations recommends that stations are placed approximately every 5 km, however, many races include more frequent stations which may influence athletes' drinking strategies and behaviors. Slower athletes with lower sweat rates, who compete in such events, particularly over prolonged distances or duration, are often able to drink in volumes that exceed their true fluid losses and are at particular risk of developing hyponatremia. Athletes taking part in these events should be educated on the importance of fluid balance and the prevention of hyperhydration. It should also be noted that in many events lasting up to 45 min, the risk of dehydration is low due to the limited duration across which sweat losses can accumulate. For faster and/or more competitive athletes, extra elements related to drinking while performing continuous exercise must be taken into consideration. This includes considerations around gastrointestinal comfort when fluid consumed during higher-intensity and "gut joggling" activities (e.g., high-speed running vs. the more "gliding" movements of cross-country skiing or cycling). Furthermore, the time lost in slowing down or moving out of an aerodynamic position to obtain or consume a drink must be factored into the overall race performance. This creates different factors in the cost: benefit analysis of an individual's fluid intake plan.

The official rules and competition characteristics of "stop-start" sports such as team and racket sports create other influences, and often unique scenarios, around fluid availability. In some examples (e.g., soccer, rugby), governing rules limit the availability of fluids for athletes during competition. Soccer, for example, includes two 45-min halves (with a continuous running clock) in which fluid availability are extremely limited to players. At the other end of the spectrum are sports such as baseball, basketball and tennis with frequent rest breaks within playing time (e.g., time outs, change of ends or player rotations) during which fluids can be consumed. An athlete's drinking strategy for a competition represents a unique instance for their particular sport based on their ability to rehydrate within the rules. We support recent governing body rule changes and referee decisions to add breaks to competitions (Major League Soccer, FIFA soccer matches, US Open Tennis) to facilitate safe participation by the athletes. These changes likely augment athletic performance and safety simultaneously. Individuals should understand their sport and its fluid needs/fluid availability characteristics to prepare and practice optimal fluid plans for competition. Where rule changes, or alterations are allowed, individuals and teams should attempt to ask for these alterations (e.g., extended rest periods, additional breaks) in advance to formulate an appropriate drinking strategy. In all sports, athletes should aim to practice and fine-tune their personal drinking strategy for race/competition conditions. This will help individuals to confirm its feasibility, understand their personal responses and develop any necessary behavioral practices within the expected rules of competition.

We define fluid availability into three distinct categories, based on particular sport variations. Sports were categorized as having high fluid availability if there are multiple opportunities for fluid consumption, rather than only during breaks. Low fluid availability was used to describe those activities involving governing rules, time constraints, or an inability to carry personal fluids during competition. Accessibility to fluid consumption during competition represents a major variable to be used in preparation of an optimal fluid replacement strategy. Practical Solutions:

- During training, ensure that there is ample access to fluids that are palatable to athletes.
- Investigate or understand the opportunities for fluid intake during that are specific to a sport or event, and any other practical issues that determine fluid intake.
- Consider the risks of hyperhydration as well as hypohydration for any sporting event or individual athlete, and prepare appropriate practice and education strategies.
- Develop personalized fluid intake plans that incorporate fluid availability characteristics of the sport or event. Where there is a likelihood of hypohydration, be proactive and creative in making use of existing opportunities for fluid intake within sport rules and characteristics and be prepared to request for changes when there is a likelihood of a serious mismatch between fluid losses and the opportunity to address these.
- Practice intended competition drinking plans ahead of time to determine their suitability and allow time for readjustment.

Intrinsic Factors

A number of intrinsic factors modulate the individual variances that are observed in fluid losses. One of the greatest considerations for an individual's sweat rate is his or her body size. Larger individuals typically have higher sweat losses, with football linemen exhibiting some of the highest recorded sweat rates. Therefore, required absolute drink volumes will be higher for these athletes. An individual's thirst drive also dictates how much they desire to drink during exercise, but this may not match their actual fluid needs. Athletes voluntarily dehydrate during exercise due to discrepancies in fluid losses and drinking behavior. Case studies of individuals who have developed hyponatremia due to excessive drinking during exercise also note that they reported thirst as an underlying contributor to their fluid intake.

Heat acclimatization contributes to variations in an individual's sweating rate responses. Individuals who are heat acclimatized exhibit greater sweat rates which can pose a greater risk of hypohydration. Although the increased sweat provides extra heat dissipation, it also requires extra fluid intake.

Women may be at greater risk for exercise-induced hyponatremia. This risk has been attributed to their lower body weight and size, excess water ingestion, and longer racing times relative to men. The greater incidence of hyponatremia in women is unlikely due to their greater levels of estradiol in plasma and tissue. Although female sex-hormones can also influence neural and hormonal control of thirst, fluid intake, sodium appetite and sodium regulation, there is no evidence that anything beyond stature and drinking behavior significantly impact their risk. Practical Solutions:

- Consider body size, acclimatization status and thirst drive when developing hydration plans for individual athletes.

Sport-Specific Factors

Weight Division, Acrobatic and Appearance-Based Sports

The culture and normal behaviors surrounding specific sports can greatly affect the hydration practices of its athletes. The three most prominent examples of the cultural effects of sports on hydration practices are weight division sports, acrobatic sports and appearance-based sports. In weight division sports (e.g., combat sports, horse racing, lightweight rowing, etc.), the practice of deliberately dehydrating to manipulate body mass to meet lighter competition weight classifications is common. In many cases, athletes not only sacrifice their performance through these practices but also endanger their health and well-being. In a similar fashion, sports where body-image and appearance are emphasized (e.g., cheerleading, body building and gymnastics), dangerous practices, such as extreme fluid restriction may be used by athletes to cheat "unofficial" weight checks that are self-instigated or expected within their training environment. Finally, "acrobatic" feats such as gymnastics, jumping and climbing are aided by a high power to weight ratio, but should not rely on severe hypohydration to achieve this. Excessive use of dehydration to manage body mass goals should be corrected to avoid long-term health complications. Practical Solutions:

- Promote healthy weight management strategies in weight division, acrobatic and appearance-based sports that minimize manipulation of body water.

Dehydration

Many athletes dehydrate during competitive events, especially long ones, even when it's not particularly hot. You can't rely on feeling thirsty as a reminder to replace fluid lost through sweating – one of nature's dirty tricks is that exercise suppresses thirst. Dehydration impairs both physical and mental performance in all types and levels of sport, yet it can be avoided (or at least minimised) by appropriate drinking strategies.

Exercise produces heat. Prevention of overheating occurs by transfer of heat to the skin by vasodilation of the cutaneous circulation, and by the cooling effect of evaporation of sweat. Exercise causes body fluid losses from moisture in exhaled air as well as from sweating. Although sweat rates are highest under conditions of high-intensity exercise in heat and high humidity, total fluid losses can be appreciable in very prolonged events, whatever the conditions. Unless fluid losses are replaced by drinks, sweating causes progressive depletion of circulating blood volume, leading to hypohydration (commonly called dehydration) and a thickening of blood. This places a strain on the cardiovascular system, with a rise in heart rate in order to maintain adequate blood flow to exercising muscles and vital organs. As blood volume depletes, blood flow to the skin is reduced. As a result, sweating decreases and heat dissipation from the skin is impaired, causing body core temperature to rise, potentially leading to heat stress, collapse and even death.

Even low levels of dehydration have physiological consequences. A loss of 2% bodyweight (just 1kg for a 50kg person) causes an increase in perceived effort and is claimed to reduce performance by 10-20% A fluid loss exceeding 3-5% bodyweight reduces aerobic exercise performance noticeably and impairs reaction time, judgment, concentration and decision making – vital elements in all sports, from pole-vaulting to football. A particular issue for boxers is that dehydration increases risk of brain injury.

The two main factors influencing early fatigue and impaired performance (both physical and mental) in all types of sports and exercise are depletion of body levels of carbohydrate (CHO) and/or fluid. Maintaining adequate CHO and fluid intake optimizes training benefit by enabling athletes to train harder and for longer, and can make a difference between winning and losing. The opportunity and ability to eat and drink during training and competition depends on the sport; sports drinks may not be the only feasible option but most of them do provide a convenient supply of CHO and fluid simultaneously, are well tolerated if used appropriately, and can be adapted to suit individual needs in varying circumstances.

There are guidelines for fluid and CHO requirements of various activities, but deciding what, when and how much an individual athlete should consume is not always straightforward. In particular, sweat rates vary among individuals subjected to the same exercise conditions. Probably the most important feature of any sports drink is PALATABILITY (in large volumes, not just a sip). The perfect drink has no value if it tastes awful, and what suits one person may not suit another.

Sweat Losses

Most research has focused on high-intensity or prolonged exercise in the heat, for obvious reasons; dehydration is potentially fatal. Sweat rate rises with exercise intensity, and is increased by a hot or humid environment and heavy clothing (notably non-whicking, dark-coloured garments), both of which interfere with heat dissipation and sweat evaporation.

Prediction of fluid and sodium (Na) losses in sweat is complicated, since sweat rates and sweat Na concentrations vary widely among individuals exercising under the same conditions. For example, measures of sweat rates during one hour of exercise at 70% VO2max at an ambient temperature fo 23 deg. C have been quoted to vary between 426g and 1665g. A study of tennis players reported sweat rates of 0.7-1.4 litres per hour among women and 1.2-2.5 litres per hour among men in hot, humid conditions (32 deg. C with a relative humidity of 60%). Absolute sweat volume is relatively less for a small, lean athlete. Training status and degree of heat-acclimatization influence composition of and volume of sweat by inducing earlier onset of sweating, a higher sweat rate and a more dilute sweat, conserving salt. Sweat Na concentration has been reported to vary between 40 and 140mmol/litre in volunteer runners, but little more than 20mmol/litre in heat-acclimatized tennis players.

Whatever the environmental conditions, sweat losses are probably greater than many athletes appreciate. The highest reported sweat rate is 3.7 litres/hour for Alberto Salazar during the 1984 Olympic marathon. Sweat rates of 2 to 3 litres/hour can be expected during short periods of hard exercise in the heat, and an excess of 1.5-2 litres/hour during endurance events. Even in cooler conditions losses are appreciable. During a football game on a cool day (10°C), players can lose up to two litres of sweat, and runners are estimated to lose around 1.2 litres/hour at 6 minute/mile pace on a cool, dry day (double this amount on a hot, humid day). Additionally, fluid is lost via moisture in exhaled air.

Except in extreme circumstances, blood Na levels are maintained during exercise. Sweat is mainly composed of water, and Na losses in sweat represent a small fraction of total body content and are readily replaced afterwards by normal food. Rare cases of hyponatraemia (blood Na depletion) have been observed, usually in events lasting eight hours or more, such as the Hawaii Ironman. This potentially life-threatening state results from 'water intoxication' – the consumption of large volumes of water or drinks containing little or no Na, or insufficient Na to match the losses in sweat which, in hot conditions over many hours, add up.

CHO-electrolyte Drinks and Performance

Since 1984, when the American College of Sports Medicine stated that water was the optimal drink for endurance exercise, many studies have shown performance-enhancing benefits of adding electrolytes (the only useful one being sodium, to speed fluid absorption) and CHO (to provide fuel).

Drinking plain water causes bloating, suppresses thirst (and thus further drinking) and stimulates urine output (therefore is inefficiently retained) – a poor choice where high fluid intake is required. Sports drinks generally contain 10-25 mmol/liter sodium, as salt – well below the optimal concentration for stimulating fluid absorption, but the ideal concentration would taste like sea-water, and palatability is vital. Optimum CHO concentration depends on the physiological demands of the sport, environmental conditions and the athlete's tolerance. In endurance sports, CHO depletion is a factor in early fatigue, but if sweat rates are high and dehydration is rapid, then fluid replacement takes priority over CHO. Powdered sports-drink formulas are practical since they can be diluted to suit the climate and the individual. Isotonic CHO-electrolyte drinks generally contain 4-8% CHO, are rapidly absorbed (as quickly as or quicker than water) and provide fuel. The benefits of CHO drinks in delaying fatigue are well documented; endurance cyclists and marathon runners achieve significantly faster times if they drink CHO-electrolyte drink in place of water and, in strength training, more reps of a given weight can be performed when CHO is consumed. This is not surprising, since the higher the exercise intensity, the more rapid the rate of CHO utilization and the sooner that glycogen stores are depleted. The results of a recent study, well-designed to mimic the physiological demands of multi-sprint sports such as football, tennis and hockey, suggest that CHO supplementation benefits both physical and mental performance tasks. In other words, CHO not only delays fatigue but also helps maintain mental alertness and judgment.

Amount of CHO

Given these finding, it seems logical to advise that CHO-electrolyte drinks are taken during endurance events and team sports alike, when food is neither practical nor manageable. But what about CHO concentration? E.F. Coyle advises, for a 68 kg man, the provision of between 30 and 60g CHO/hour in the form of between 625 and 1250 ml/hour of a 4-8% CHO-electrolyte drink during endurance exercise. (Quantities should obviously be adjusted for different body weights.) In reality, however, some athletes find a 4-8% CHO drink 'heavy' and choose a weaker solution for easier tolerance, although tolerance of CHO drinks during exercise does improve with practice. In ultra-events in the heat, where large volumes (usually 1-1.4 litres/hour) are recommended, boredom and flavour-fatigue can be a problem, in which case, a choice of drinks and the option of CHO-containing foods (if tolerated) can help.

In most sports situations, drinks in excess of 10% CHO concentration are inadvisable. However, during prolonged (more than 60-90 minutes) high-intensity exercise in very cold conditions, with low sweat rates, glycogen depletion is more a factor than dehydration, and a drink with up to 15% may be more beneficial, if tolerated.

Many endurance athletes incur a deficit of fluid and CHO during competition. Sandwiches and tumblers of squash would help to replenish body stores, but post-event loss of appetite is common. CHO-electrolyte drinks may be easier to manage, are rapidly absorbed, well retained and relatively easy to drink in quantity since their sodium content drives thirst. For these reasons, CHO-electrolyte drinks can be particularly valuable in multi-stage events such as, for example, the Tour de France, major tennis tournaments and two-day mountain marathons, where not only are CHO and fluid requirements high but there is limited time to refuel and rehydrate before the next day. In these situations, even athletes with huge appetites may have difficulty replenishing glycogen stores with food alone in the time available, and CHO-electrolyte drinks can be a useful top-up.

Reason of Dehydration in Athletes

Dehydration is progressive depletion of body fluids caused when fluid losses, for whatever reason, exceed fluid intake. This leads to hypohydration (or dehydration). Athletes may arrive at the start of their event already hypo hydrated – for example, after a long, hot journey to the event, or inadequate rehydration in between successive events, or 'making weight' strategies in, for instance, boxing, light-weight rowing and horseracing. Possible reasons for insufficient fluid intake during an event include:

- Poor understanding of fluid requirements: Because sweat rates vary so widely and are probably greater than most athletes appreciate, a worthwhile plan is to record fluid intake during training or events (also noting the weather conditions) and weighing, without clothes, before and after, to assess how well fluid intake matches losses.

- Limited opportunity to drink, or availability of drinks: Orienteers and fell runners common carry little or no drink, relying instead on streams. For events lasting an hour or more, if the availability of streams cannot be guaranteed, consumption of 500 ml of an electrolyte, or CHO-electrolyte, drink 10 minutes before the start will benefit performance in later stages.

- Poor drinking strategies: As I've said, exercise suppresses thirst, and the event itself can distract the athlete from drinking. Subsequent hypohydration impairs gastric emptying and can cause gastric upset, nausea or vomiting, which in turn limit further ability to drink.

- Poor tolerance of drinks during competition: The nausea that many athletes blame on sports drinks could be caused by dehydration itself, or too concentrated a drink. Dehydration can be mistaken for carbohydrate depletion. Drinks that contain more than 10% CHO impair gastric emptying (and therefore rate of fluid provision) and stimulate the secretion of body fluids into the intestine to dilute the drink before it can be absorbed, temporarily worsening dehydration.
- High CHO drinks can themselves cause nausea, more so in a dehydrated athlete. Carbonated drinks are likely to cause bloating or discomfort, and fructose (fruit sugar) in high concentrations can cause gastric upset and/or diarrhoea. Although fructose is included in some sports drinks, it is inefficient as a sole source of CHO because it is absorbed slowly and requires conversion to glucose by the liver before it is available for energy.
- Inability to match excessive sweat rates: Exercise intensities exceeding 70% VO-2max will progressively suppress gastric emptying. The highest reported rate of gastric emptying is 2400ml/hour, in resting subjects. During exercise gastric emptying rarely exceeds 1-1.2 litres/hour, unless a large volume is maintained in the stomach. Runners in particular experience discomfort with high volumes in the stomach, and in race situations it is unlikely that athletes could drink more than two litres/hour, even if they could tolerate it. Some degree of dehydration is therefore inevitable when rates of fluid loss exceed sustainable drinking capacity.

In practice, competing endurance runners and canoeists generally drink about 500 ml/hour, and dehydrate at a rate of 500-1000 ml/hour. Even triathletes, who as a group are relatively knowledgeable about nutrition and hydration, have been shown to lose an average of 1.7% and 3.7% of bodyweight for a 3-hour and a 12-hour event respectively. Whereas cyclists are known to tolerate 1.2 litres/hour of a 6% CHO-electrolyte drink, runners are more likely to experience discomfort, and may believe that time lost through slowing down to drink may not be recovered. The volume that most athletes choose to drink during exercise replaces less than 50% of their losses. With this in mind, effective post-event hydration is vital in between consecutive heats or events spanning several days.

References

- Principle-caloric-balance-7200: healthyeating.sfgate.com, Retrieved 22, March 2020
- Energy-balance-in-sport-and-the-three-goals, nutrition: maximuscle.com, Retrieved 10, June 2020
- All-about-energy-balance: precisionnutrition.com, Retrieved 09, August 2020
- Dehydration-sport-vital-athlete-maintains-hydration-levels-exercise, fuelling-and-hydration-for-exercise, nutrition-for-endurance-athletes: peakendurancesport.com, , Retrieved 25, 2020
- Importance-of-hydration: hydralytesports.com.au, Retrievedo 2, July 2020
- Energy-requirements-for-athletes, michael-long-nd: ontariohealth.org, Retrieved 25, May 2020

3

Types of Dietary Supplements

Dietary supplements are products taken orally as a supplement to a regular diet for the sole purpose of providing additional nutrients to the body. They usually contain one or more ingredients such as vitamins or amino acids. Energy bars, sports drinks, energy gels, diet drinks, etc. are all forms of dietary supplements. This chapter has been carefully written to provide an easy understanding of the subject matter.

Dietary Supplement

Flight through a CT image stack of a multivitamin tablet "A-Z" by German company Abtei.

A dietary supplement is intended to provide nutrients that may otherwise not be consumed in sufficient quantities.

Supplements as generally understood include vitamins, minerals, fiber, fatty acids, or amino acids, among other substances. U.S. authorities define dietary supplements as foods, while elsewhere they may be classified as drugs or other products.

There are more than 50,000 dietary supplements available. More than half of the U.S. adult population (53% - 55%) consume dietary supplements with most common ones being multivitamins.

These products are not intended to prevent or treat any disease and in some circumstances are dangerous, according to the U.S. National Institutes of Health. For those who fail to consume a balanced diet, the agency says that certain supplements "may have value."

Most supplements should be avoided, and usually people should not eat micronutrients except people with clearly shown deficiency. Those people should first consult a doctor. An exception is vitamin D, which is recommended in Nordic countries due to weak sunlight.

Definition

According to the United States Food and Drug Administration (FDA), dietary supplements are products which are not pharmaceutical drugs, food additives like spices or preservatives, or conventional food, and which also meet any of these criteria.

1. The product is intended to supplement a person's diet, despite it not being usable as a meal replacement.

2. The product is or contains a vitamin, dietary element, herb used for herbalism or botanical used as a medicinal plant, amino acid, any substance which contributes to other food eaten, or any concentrate, metabolite, ingredient, extract, or combination of these things.

3. The product is labeled as a dietary supplement.

In the United States, the FDA has different monitoring procedures for substances depending on whether they are presented as drugs, food additives, food, or dietary supplements. Dietary supplements are eaten or taken by mouth, and are regulated in United States law as a type of food rather than a type of drug. Like food and unlike drugs, no government approval is required to make or sell dietary supplements; the manufacturer checks the safety of dietary supplements but the government does not; and rather than requiring risk–benefit analysis to prove that the product can be sold like a drug, risk–benefit analysis is only used to petition that food or a dietary supplement is unsafe and should be removed from market.

Medical Uses

The intended use of dietary supplements is to ensure that a person gets enough essential nutrients.

Dietary supplements should not be used to treat any disease or as preventive healthcare. An exception to this recommendation is the appropriate use of vitamins.

Dietary supplements are unnecessary if one eats a balanced diet.

Supplements may create harm in several ways, including over-consumption, particularly of minerals and fat-soluble vitamins which can build up in the body. The products may also cause harm related to their rapid absorption in a short period of time, quality issues such as contamination, or by adverse interactions with other foods and medications.

Vitamins

Vitamin is an organic compound required by an organism as a vital nutrient in limited amounts. An organic chemical compound (or related set of compounds) is called a vitamin when it cannot be synthesized in sufficient quantities by an organism, and must be obtained from the diet. Thus, the term is conditional both on the circumstances and on the particular organism. For example, ascorbic acid (vitamin C) is a vitamin for humans, but not for most other animals. Supplementation is important for the treatment of certain health problems but there is little evidence of benefit when used by those who are otherwise healthy.

Types

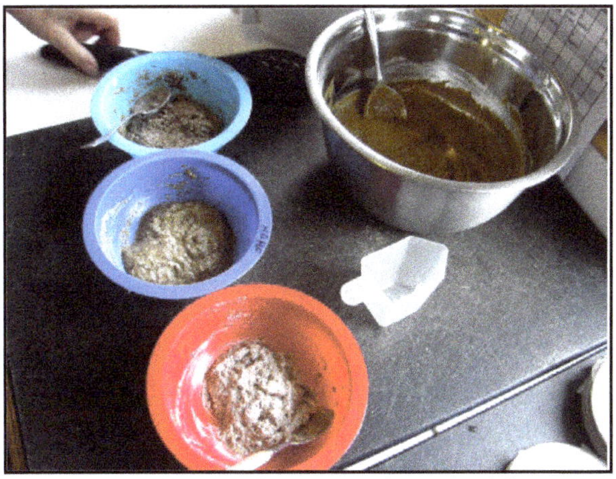

Dietary supplements being mixed into food for pigs.

Dietary Element

Dietary elements, commonly called "dietary minerals" or "minerals", are the chemical elements required by living organisms, other than the four elements carbon, hydrogen, nitrogen, and oxygen present in common organic molecules. The term "dietary mineral" is archaic, as the substances it refers are chemical elements rather than actual minerals.

Herbal Medicine

Herbal medicine is the use of plants for medicinal purposes. Plants have been the basis for medical treatments through much of human history, and such traditional medicine is still widely practiced today. Modern medicine recognizes herbalism as a form of alternative medicine, as the practice of herbalism is not strictly based on evidence gathered using the scientific method. Modern medicine, does, however, make use of many plant-derived compounds as the basis for evidence-tested pharmaceutical drugs, and phytotherapy works to apply modern standards of effectiveness testing to herbs and medicines that are derived from natural sources. The scope of herbal medicine is sometimes extended to include fungal and bee products, as well as minerals, shells and certain animal parts.

Amino Acids and Proteins

Amino acids are biologically important organic compounds composed of amine ($-NH_2$) and carboxylic acid (-COOH) functional groups, along with a side-chain specific to each amino acid. The key elements of an amino acid are carbon, hydrogen, oxygen, and nitrogen, though other elements are found in the side-chains of certain amino acids.

Amino acids can be divided into three categories: essential amino acids, non-essential amino acids, and conditional amino acids. Essential amino acids cannot be made by the body, and must be supplied by food. Non-essential amino acids are made by the body from essential amino acids or in the normal breakdown of proteins. Conditional amino acids are usually not essential, except in times of illness, stress, or for someone challenged with a lifelong medical condition.

Essential Fatty Acids

Essential fatty acids, or EFAs, are fatty acids that humans and other animals must ingest because the body requires them for good health but cannot synthesize them. The term "essential fatty acid" refers to fatty acids required for biological processes but does not include the fats that only act as fuel.

Bodybuilding Supplements

Bodybuilding supplements are dietary supplements commonly used by those involved in bodybuilding and athletics. Bodybuilding supplements may be used to replace meals, enhance weight gain, promote weight loss or improve athletic performance. Among the most widely used are vitamin supplements, protein drinks, branched-chain amino acids (BCAA), glutamine, essential fatty acids, meal replacement products, creatine, weight loss products and testosterone boosters. Supplements are sold either as single ingredient preparations or in the form of "stacks" – proprietary blends of various supplements marketed as offering synergistic advantages. While many bodybuilding supplements are also consumed by the general public their salience and frequency of use may differ when used specifically by bodybuilders.

Industry

In 2013, the global market of vitamins, minerals, and nutritional and herbal supplements (VMHS) was valued at $82 billion, with roughly 28 percent of that in the U.S., where sales increased by approximately $6 billion between 2007 and 2012.

The vitamins and dietary supplements sector in the U.S. grew 4% in 2015, to reach US$27.2 billion. The U.S. market was highly competitive in 2015, as no single company accounted for more than a 5% share of value sales.

Controversy

According to University of Helsinki food safety professor Marina Heinonen, more than 90% of dietary supplement health claims are incorrect. In addition, ingredients listed have been found to be different from the contents. For example, Consumer Reports reported unsafe levels of arsenic, cadmium, lead and mercury in several of the protein powders that were tested. Also, the CBC found that protein spiking (the addition of amino acid filler to manipulate analysis) was not uncommon, however many of the companies involved challenged their claim.

Adverse Effects

The number of incidents of liver damage from dietary supplements has tripled in a decade. Most of the products causing that effect were bodybuilding supplements. Some of the victims required liver transplants and some died. A third of the supplements involved contained unlisted steroids.

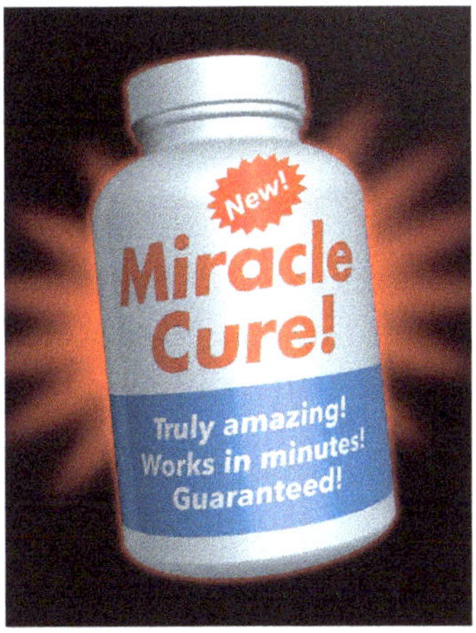

Some products make extraordinary claims and contain active ingredients which may not have been proven effective.

Mild to severe toxicity has occurred on many occasions due to dietary supplements, even when the active ingredients were essential nutrients such as vitamins, minerals or amino acids. This has been a result of adulteration of the product, excessive usage on the part of the consumer, or use by persons at risk for the development of adverse effects. In addition, a number of supplements contain psychoactive drugs, whether of natural or synthetic origin.

Physical and Chemical Properties

Adulteration in North America

BMC Medicine published a study on herbal supplements in 2013. Most of the supplements studied were of low quality, one third did not contain the active ingredient(s) claimed, and one third contained unlisted substances.

An investigation by the New York Attorney General's office reported in 2015 analyzed 78 bottles of herbal supplements from Walmart, Target, Walgreens and GNC stores in New York State using DNA barcoding, a method used to detect labeling fraud in the seafood industry. Only about 20% contained the ingredient on the label.

Some supplements were contamined by rodent feces and urine.

Only 0.3% of the 55,000 U.S. market dietary supplements have been studied regarding their common side effects.

Society and Culture

Public Health

Work done by scientists in the early 20th century on identifying individual nutrients in food and developing ways to manufacture them raised hopes that optimal health could be achieved and diseases prevented by adding them to food and providing people with dietary supplements; while there were successes in preventing vitamin deficiencies, and preventing conditions like neural tube defects by supplementation and food fortification with folic acid, no targeted supplementation or fortification strategies to prevent major diseases like cancer or cardiovascular diseases have proved successful.

For example, while increased consumption of fruits and vegetables are related to decreases in mortality, cardiovascular diseases and cancers, supplementation with key factors found in fruits and vegetable, like antioxidants, vitamins, or minerals, do not help and some have been found to be harmful in some cases. In general as of 2016, robust clinical data is lacking, that shows that any kind of dietary supplementation does more good than harm for people who are healthy and eating a reasonable diet but there is clear data showing that dietary pattern and lifestyle choices are associated with health outcomes.

As a result of the lack of good data for supplementation and the strong data for dietary pattern, public health recommendations for healthy eating urge people to eat a plant-based diet of whole foods, minimizing processed food, salt and sugar and to get exercise daily, and to abandon Western pattern diets and a sedentary lifestyle.

Legal Regulation

United States

The regulation of food and dietary supplements by the U.S. Food and Drug Administration is governed by various statutes enacted by the United States Congress and interpreted by the U.S. Food and Drug Administration ("FDA"). Pursuant to the Federal Food, Drug, and Cosmetic Act ("the Act") and accompanying legislation, the FDA has authority to oversee the quality of substances sold as food in the United States, and to monitor claims made in the labeling about both the composition and the health benefits of foods.

Substances which the FDA regulates as food are subdivided into various categories, including foods, food additives, added substances (man-made substances which are not intentionally introduced into food, but nevertheless end up in it), and dietary supplements. The specific standards which the FDA exercises differ from one category to the next. Furthermore, the FDA has been granted a variety of means by which it can address violations of the standards for a given category of substances.

Regulation in European Union

The European Union's Food Supplements Directive of 2002 requires that supplements be demonstrated to be safe, both in dosages and in purity. Only those supplements that have been proven to be safe may be sold in the bloc without prescription. As a category of food, food supplements cannot be labeled with drug claims but can bear health claims and nutrition claims.

The dietary supplements industry in the United Kingdom (UK), one of the 28 countries in the bloc, strongly opposed the Directive. In addition, a large number of consumers throughout Europe, including over one million in the UK, and various doctors and scientists, had signed petitions by 2005 against what are viewed by the petitioners as unjustified restrictions of consumer choice.

In 2004, along with two British trade associations, the Alliance for Natural Health (ANH) had a legal challenge to the Food Supplements Directive referred to the European Court of Justice by the High Court in London.

Although the European Court of Justice's Advocate General subsequently said that the bloc's plan to tighten rules on the sale of vitamins and food supplements should be scrapped, he was eventually overruled by the European Court, which decided that the measures in question were necessary and appropriate for the purpose of protecting public health. ANH, however, interpreted the ban as applying only to synthetically produced supplements—and not to vitamins and minerals normally found in or consumed as part of the diet.

Nevertheless, the European judges acknowledged the Advocate General's concerns, stating that there must be clear procedures to allow substances to be added to the permitted list based on scientific evidence. They also said that any refusal to add the product to the list must be open to challenge in the courts.

Research

Effects of most dietary supplements have not been determined in randomized clinical trials and manufacturing is lightly regulated; randomized clinical trials of certain vitamins and antioxidants have found increased mortality rates.

Energy Bar

Energy bars are supplemental bars containing cereals and other high energy foods targeted at people who require quick energy but do not have time for a meal. They are different from energy drinks, which contain caffeine, whereas bars provide food energy.

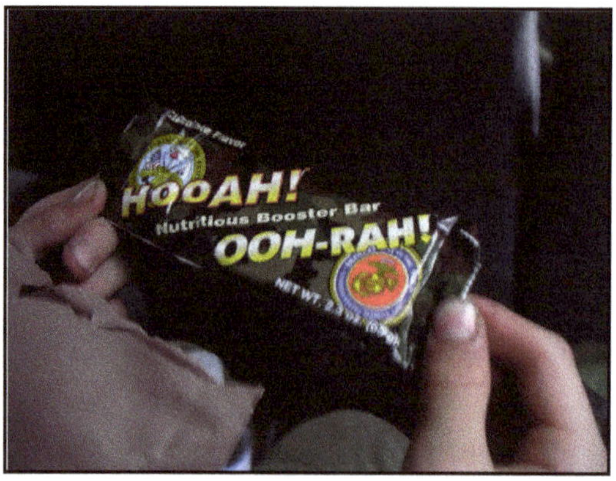

A HOOAH! energy bar provided by the United States Army in its MREs.

Nutrition

Energy in food comes from all three main sources: fat, protein, and carbohydrates. A typical energy bar weighs between 45 and 80 g and is likely to supply about 200–300 Cal (840–1,300 kJ), 3–9 g of fat, 7–15 g of protein, and 20–40 g of carbohydrates.

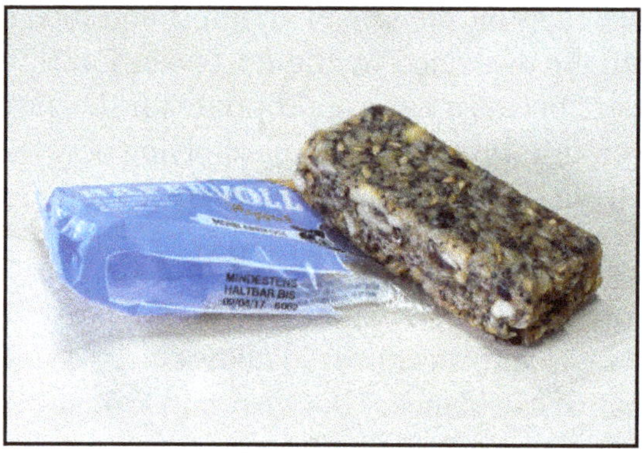

Full Flapjack bars.

In order to provide energy quickly, most of the carbohydrates are various types of sugars like fructose, glucose, maltodextrin, dextrose and others in various ratios. Use of complex carbohydrate sources like oats and barley is limited and such carbohydrate sources are mostly used in protein bars. Proteins come mostly in the form of fast digesting whey protein. Energy bars generally don't contain sugar alcohols, since these bars, due to type of carbohydrate content, don't require low calorie sweeteners to improve their taste. Fats in energy bars are kept to minimum and their main sources are often cocoa butter and dark chocolate.

Usage

Energy bars are used as energy source during athletic events like marathon, triathlon and other events and outdoor activities, where energy expenditure is high, for longer period of time.

Sports Drink

Sports drinks are beverages whose stated purpose is to help athletes replace water, electrolytes, and energy after training or competition, though their efficacy for that purpose has been questioned, particularly after exercise.

Categories of Sport Drinks

Sports drinks can be split into three major types.

- Isotonic sport drinks contain similar concentrations of salt and sugar as in the human body.
- Hypertonic sport drinks contain a higher concentration of salt and sugar than the human body.
- Hypotonic sport drinks contain a lower concentration of salt and sugar than the human body.

Most sports drinks are approximately isotonic, having between 4 and 5 heaped teaspoons of sugar per five ounce (13 and 19 grams per 250ml) serving.

Purpose and Effectiveness

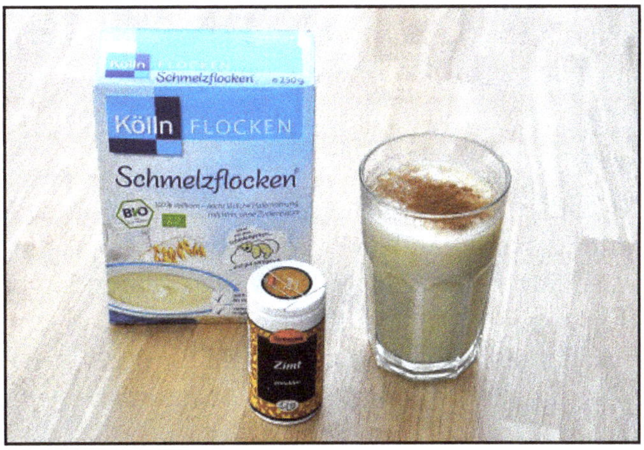

Sport drink made with processed oats, cinnamon, orange juice and milk.

Athletes actively training and competing lose water and electrolytes by sweating, and expending energy. However, Robert Robergs, an exercise physiologist at the University of New Mexico who studied Gatorade, said that unless someone is exercising or competing in a sporting event for longer than 90 minutes, there is no reason to drink something with excess sugar and electrolytes. The Australian Institute of Sport states that excessive salt supplementation during exercise may lead to "gastrointestinal problems or cause further impairment of fluid balance" and may cause salt-induced cramps.

Sodium in drinks might help to avoid hyponatraemia (low sodium), but only after sustaining athletic activity for more than four hours; a sports drink containing sodium may be appropriate for recovery from intense and prolonged training or competition.

A stated purpose of sports drinks, which provide many calories of energy from sugars, is to improve performance and endurance. In an analysis by Matthew Thompson and colleagues from the Oxford Centre for Evidence Based Medicine, of 431 marketing claims of performance enhancement, most cited no evidence. 174 sources were cited for GlaxoSmithKline's Lucozade; of them, Thompson found only three studies of high quality with a low risk of bias. The rigorous studies that did show improved endurance were "of limited relevance to most people because the tests were on elite athletes". Thompson said that, for the vast majority of people, drinking such products "could completely counteract exercising more, playing football more, going to the gym more".

The drinks are marketed as soft drinks. In response to the Oxford analysis, a soft drinks industry spokesman claimed "By helping people participating in sport to perform better and to recover more quickly, sports drinks can encourage people to exercise more".

An effect of drinking sports drinks with carbohydrates without prolonged exercise is weight gain. A study presented at the Obesity Society's Obesity 2012 scientific meeting found people in their teens gained 3.5 pounds (1.6 kg) over two years for every bottle of sports drink consumed per day. The leading author of the study, Alison Field of Harvard Medical School, said she was surprised to find that "Sports drinks have an even stronger relationship than sugared sodas with weight gain".

History

In the 19th and early 20th century, athletes occasionally drank beer of low alcohol content replenishing water, minerals and energy in the body. As the water is boiled during the brewing process and thus sterilized, the beer was safer option than water from an unknown source. However, it is studied that even a low dose of ethanol decreases endurance performance: it inhibits liver glucose output during exercise, and also impairs psychomotor skills such as reaction time, hand-eye coordination and balance.

High-protein Diet

A high-protein diet is often recommended by bodybuilders and nutritionists to help efforts to build muscle and lose fat. It should not be confused with low-carbohydrate diets, such as the Atkins Diet, which are not food-energy–controlled and which often contain large amounts of fat.

While adequate protein is required for building skeletal muscle and other tissues, there is ongoing debate regarding the use and necessity of high-protein diets in anaerobic exercise, in particular for weight training and bodybuilding.

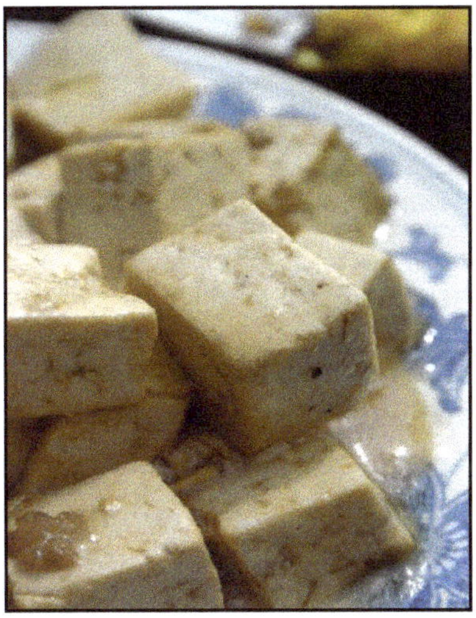

Examples of high-protein foods are tofu (shown above), dairy products, fish, and meat.

Health Effects

Extreme protein intake (in excess of 200 g per day), coupled with inadequate intake of other calorie sources (fat or carbohydrates), can cause a form of metabolic disturbance and death commonly known as rabbit starvation. Even when consuming other calorie sources, consuming more than 285 g of protein per day (for an 80 kg person) may be unsafe.

Relatively little evidence has been gathered regarding the effect of more moderate long-term high intake of protein on the development of chronic diseases. Increased load on the kidney is a result of an increase in reabsorption of NaCl. This causes a decrease in the sensitivity of tubuloglomerular feedback, which, in turn, results in an increased glomerular filtration rate. This increases pressure in glomerular capillaries. When added to any additional renal disease, this may cause permanent glomerular damage.

As is apparent from the list below, many high-protein foods (indeed, most low-carb foods with protein) are fairly low in fiber. This can lead to discomfort if additional roughage is not added to the diet.

High-protein Foods

High-protein foods include:

Food	Protein fraction by mass
Soy protein isolate	88%
Boiled green soybeans	12%[a]

Whey protein concentrate	up to 89%
Whey protein isolate	at least 90%
Peanuts	24%[b]
Steak	27 to 34%[c]
Chicken breast	31%[d]
Salmon fillet	25%[e]
Tuna (canned)	19%[f]

Protein and Weight Training

Protein is described as essential by advocates of the high-protein diet, which includes a large proportion of the bodybuilding community; it is claimed to provide the muscle with amino acids required to repair the damage done by anaerobic exercise. High protein consumption leads to increased levels of IGF-1, a hormone which, among other things, increases muscle protein synthesis. Some consume protein supplements after bodybuilding workouts, as they provide a quick and easily consumable protein source. Alternatively, meat, beans, or other high-protein foods are consumed.

It is possible to maintain a strict vegan high-protein diet, though due to the lower protein density of plant-based foods this requires a larger absolute volume of food compared to a non-vegan diet; simply put, vegans must consume a lot more food to get a lot of protein. Legumes and soy foods are two vegan sources with high protein content per calorie. Vegans may engage in protein combining to obtain a complete mix of amino acids.

Although some testing shows that the body will absorb and use a greater amount of protein after "bodybuilding" type exercises than under more sedentary circumstances, and some studies on weight training show clinically significant gains in muscle with a very high protein diet when compared to more moderate intake, in some studies increased protein intake fails to translate into functional differences in strength or muscle size. However, consistently consuming less protein than an individual's body requires (approximately 0.7g/kg/day for a sedentary individual) causes loss of existing lean body mass, even with an excessively caloric diet.

Energy Gel

Energy gels are carbohydrate gels that provide energy for exercise and promote recovery, commonly used in endurance events such as running, cycling, and triathlons. Energy gels are also referred to as endurance gels, sports gels, nutritional gels, and carbohydrate gels. They come in small, single-serve plastic packets. Each packet has a strip with a small notch at the top that can be peeled off to reveal an opening through which the gel can be consumed.

History

Sports energy gels emerged in the United Kingdom in 1986 as a "convenient, pre-wrapped, portable" way to deliver carbohydrates during endurance events. Gels have a gooey texture and are sometimes referred to as "goo" generically. The gel Leppin Squeezy was distributed at the Hawaii Ironman Triathlon in 1988. Once considered a "cult product in clear packaging", energy gel products are now marketed in fancy packaging and come in a variety of flavors. The energy gel market grew during the 1990s, as professional athletes began endorsing products. Manufacturers generally encourage the consumption of multiple packets, with water, when participating in endurance events. Individual packets typically cost between 99 cents and $1.29 (as reported by the *St. Petersburg Times* in 2003).

Nutritional Behavior

Once consumed, the carbohydrates found in the gels are absorbed into the blood to supply the body with calories and nutrients to fuel exercise activity by helping to delay muscular fatigue, raise blood sugar levels, and enhance performance. Most energy gels have no fat, fiber, or protein, so they can be digested quickly. They contain mainly sugars and maltodextrins, which make them similar to sports drinks without the water. Some gels, such as e-Gel, also come with added electrolytes. There are also gels with extras such as ginseng and other herbs, amino acids, vitamins, and Coenzyme Q10. Caffeine can be found in some gels as well. Examples of common energy gels are GU, PowerBar Gel, and Clif Shot.

Use

The recommended use of an energy gel is 15 minutes before starting and 30–45 minutes after starting the endurance exercise. The first gel prior to exercise may be skipped in favor of a high carbohydrate snack instead. Energy gels are then to be used every 30–45 minutes during exercise. The notch can be peeled off at the top and an intake of energy gel is recommended to be followed with a drink of water to avoid risk of dehydration. The exact intake of the gel varies for every athlete depending on their metabolism, body weight, and fitness level.

Diet Drink

Diet (alternatively marketed as sugar-free, zero-calorie or low-calorie) drinks are sugar-free, artificially sweetened versions of fizzy beverages with virtually no calories. They are generally marketed toward health-conscious people, diabetics, athletes, and other people who want to lose weight, improve physical fitness, or reduce their sugar intake.

History

The beginning of the diet drink or refreshment era was in 1952, when Kirsch Bottling in Brooklyn, New York launched a sugar-free ginger ale called No-Cal. It was designed for diabetics, not dieters, and distribution remained local. Royal Crown Cola placed an announcement in an Atlanta newspaper in 1958 announcing a diet product, Diet Rite. In 1962, Dr Pepper released a diet(etic) version of its soft drink, although it sold slowly due to the misconception that it was meant solely for diabetic consumption. In 1963, The Coca-Cola Company joined the diet soft drink market with Tab, which proved to be a huge success. Tab was originally sweetened with cyclamates and saccharin.

Tab, Diet Rite, and Fresca (a grapefruit-flavored drink introduced by Coca-Cola) were the only brand-name diet refreshments on the market until Pepsi released Patio Diet Cola in 1963 and renamed Diet Pepsi the following year. Diet 7 Up was released in 1963 under the name Like. It was discontinued in 1969 due to the U.S. government ban of cyclamate sweetener. After reformulation, it was reintroduced as Diet 7 Up in 1970. It was renamed Sugar Free 7 Up in 1973 then back to Diet 7 Up in 1979. Coca-Cola countered by releasing Diet Coke in 1982. After the release of Diet Coke, Tab took a backseat on the Coca-Cola production lines; Diet Coke could be more easily identified by consumers as associated with Coca-Cola than Tab. Additionally, a study was released claiming that saccharin was a possible carcinogen, leading to Coca-Cola's decision to decrease production of Tab. Prompted by the rising popularity of soft drinks, in the mid-1980s some of those in the alcohol industry began to follow their lead with some beer companies putting sugar-free beer on the market.

By the early 1990s, a wide array of companies had their own diet refreshments on supermarket shelves. Tab made a comeback during the late 1990s, after new studies demonstrated that saccharin is not an important factor in the risk of cancer. Nevertheless, The Coca-Cola Company has maintained its 1984 reformulation, replacing some of the saccharin in Tab with NutraSweet.

By 2002, some beverage companies had diversified to include such flavors as vanilla and lemon among their products, and diet drinks were soon being produced with those flavors as well. By 2004, several alcohol companies had released sugar-free or "diet" alcoholic products too.

Sweetening

Multiple artificial sweeteners can be used to give diet soft drinks a sweet taste without sugar. Sometimes two sweeteners are used in the same beverage. Opinion is mixed as to the taste of these beverages: some think they lack the taste of their sugar-sweetened counterparts, while others think the taste is similar. Some also note an unusual non-sugary aftertaste. Some[t] feel the opposite—that diet drinks have no aftertaste and that drinks sweetened by high fructose corn syrup have a gritty, over-sweet aftertaste.

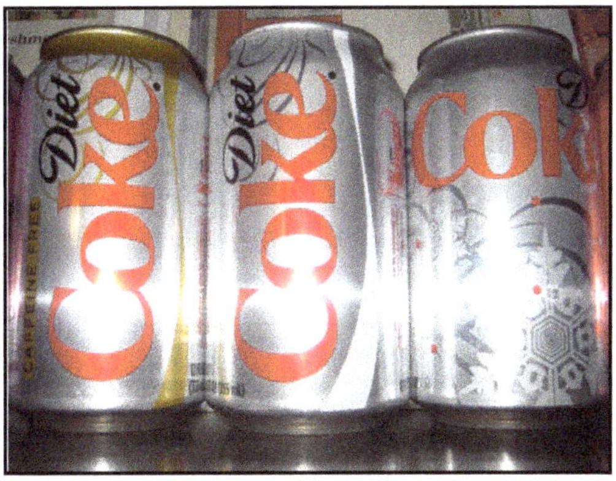

Diet Coke is the number one selling diet soft drink in the world.

Aspartame

Aspartame, commonly known by the brand name NutraSweet, is one of the most commonly used artificial sweeteners. The 1982 introduction of aspartame-sweetened Diet Coke accelerated this trend. Today, at least in the United States, "diet" is nearly synonymous with the use of aspartame in beverages.

Cyclamates

The first artificial sweeteners used in diet soft drinks were cyclamates (often synergistically with saccharin). While many say these cyclamate-sweetened beverages had a more pleasant taste than the diet drinks that followed them, the Food and Drug Administration banned cyclamates in the United States in 1970 on evidence that they caused cancer in lab rats. Cyclamates are still used in many countries outside of the United States.

Saccharin

Once cyclamates were banned, American producers turned to saccharin. When used by itself, saccharin was often criticized for having a bitter taste and "chemical" aftertaste. Some products, such as Coca-Cola's Tab, attempted to rectify this by adding a small amount of sugar. In 1977, the FDA was petitioned to ban saccharin, too, as a carcinogen, but a moratorium was placed on the ban until studies were conducted. The ban was lifted in 1991, but by that time, virtually all diet soft drink production had shifted to using aspartame. Perhaps the most notable holdout is Tab, which also uses some aspartame in its formula.

Sucralose and Acesulfame Potassium; "Sugar-free" Soft Drinks

Recently, two other sweeteners have been used with increasing frequency: sucralose (marketed as Splenda) and acesulfame potassium ("Sunett" or "Ace K"). The K in "Ace K" represents the chemical symbol for potassium. Acesulfame potassium is usually combined with aspartame, sucralose, or saccharin rather than alone and its use is particularly common among smaller beverage producers (e.g. Big Red). Diet Rite is the non-aspartame diet soft drink brand with the highest sales today; it uses a combination of sucralose and acesulfame potassium.

Advocates say drinks employing these sweeteners have a more natural sugar-like taste than those made just with aspartame, and do not have a strong aftertaste. The newer aspartame-free drinks can also be safely consumed by phenylketonurics, because they do not contain phenylalanine. Critics say the taste is not better, merely different, or note that the long-term health risks of all or certain artificial sweeteners is unclear.

The widespread, though not universal, agreement that the newest formulations taste much more "normal" (sugar-like) than the older diet soft drinks have prompted some producers, such as Jones Soda, to abandon the "diet" label entirely in favor of "sugar-free", implying that the taste is good enough to drink even when not trying to lose weight. (This idea was first floated by Diet Coke in 1984, with the tagline, "Just For the Taste of It.")

In 2005, The Coca-Cola Company announced it would produce a sucralose-containing formulation of Diet Coke known as Diet Coke with Splenda, but that it would continue to produce the aspartame version as well. There were also rumors that a sugar-free version of Coca-Cola Classic, also sweetened with sucralose, was being formulated as well. This formulation was eventually called Coca-Cola Zero, though it is sweetened with aspartame in conjunction with acesulfame potassium.

Stevia

Initially launched in Argentina in 2013, Coca-Cola Life is made with a mix of stevia and sugar as its sweeteners. Pepsi has also released a variant of their cola sweetened with stevia and sugar, called Pepsi Next.

Amount of Artificial Sweeteners in Diet Soft Drinks

The table below displays milligrams of sweetener in an 8-ounce serving of bottled or canned soft drink as provided by the manufacturers. To determine the amount in a 12-ounce can, multiply these numbers by 1.5. Fountain drinks may contain different sweeteners or different amounts of the same sweeteners.

Beverage	Saccharin (mg)	Aspartame (mg)	Acesulfame K (mg)	Sucralose (mg)	Phosphoric Acid (mg)
Diet Coke	0	125	30	0	43
Diet Coke, caffeitne free	0	125	0	0	0
Diet Coke with Splenda	0	0	0	40	0

Coke Zero	0		58		31		38		28	
Diet Pepsi	0		111		7		0		0	
Caffeine Free Diet Pepsi	0		118		0		0		0	
Diet Pepsi Lime	0		83		21		0		0	
Diet Pepsi Vanilla	0		83		21		0		0	
Pepsi One	0		0		30		40		0	
Pepsi Max	0		77		20		0		0	
Pepsi Next	0		0		7		17		0	
Diet Dr. Pep-per	0		123		0		0		0	
Diet Mountain Dew	0		57		18		18		0	
Sprite Zero	0		50		34		0		0	
Fresca	0		50		34		0		0	
Tab	64		19		0		0		0	
Barq's Diet Root Beer	0		66		41		0		0	

Health Concerns

Many consumers are concerned about possible health effects of sugar substitutes and caffeine overuse. The effectiveness of diet soft drinks as a weight loss tool has also been called into question.

Changing the food energy intake from one food will not necessarily change a person's overall food energy intake or cause a person to lose weight. One study at the University of Texas Health Science Center at San Antonio, reported by Sharon Fowler at the ADA annual meeting, actually suggested the opposite, where consumption of diet drinks correlated with weight gain. While Fowler did suggest that the undelivered expected calories from diet drinks may stimulate the appetite, the correlation does not prove that consumption of diet drinks caused the weight gain. The ADA has yet to issue an updated policy concerning diet drinks.

In an independent study by researchers with the Framingham Heart Study in Massachusetts, consumption of any kind of soft drink correlated with increased incidence of metabolic syndrome. Of the 9,000 males and females studied, these drinkers were at 48% higher risk for metabolic syndrome, which involves weight gain and elevated blood sugar. No significant difference in these findings was observed between sugary and diet soft drinks. The researchers surmised that diet drinkers were less likely to consume healthy foods, and that drinking diet beverages flavored with artificial sweeteners more than likely increases cravings for sugar-flavored sweets.

Nomenclature

In countries outside of the United States, United Kingdom and Canada, the term "light" is often used instead of "diet"; sometimes, even in countries that do not speak English, the word "light" in English is used (e.g., "Coca-Cola Light" in Spain). The formulation of these is slightly different than the "diet"-named versions and thus the taste is slightly different.

Reduced-calorie Drinks

In an effort to profit on the surging popularity of low-carbohydrate diets, Coca-Cola and Pepsico both released reduced-calorie versions of their flagship colas in 2004. The products contain approximately half the sugar of the regular versions. The Pepsi variant, Pepsi Edge, is sweetened with sucralose and corn syrup. The sweetening of the Coca-Cola variant, Coca-Cola C2, is a combination of corn syrup, aspartame, acesulfame potassium and sucralose. Pepsi discontinued Edge in 2005, citing lackluster sales. Coca-Cola soon followed suit. Pepsi then released Pepsi Max in 2012.

Half of the sugar of a can of regular cola still exceeds the daily sugar allowance of some popular low-carbohydrate diets. It is possible that these soft drinks were targeted to so-called "carb-conscious consumers", who are paying attention to their carbohydrate intake but not trying to drastically reduce it.

Consumption

According to a study by the National Center for Health Statistics, about one-fifth of the U.S. population ages 2 years and over consumed diet drinks on a given day in 2009–2010, and 11% consumed 16 fluid oz. of diet drinks or more. Overall, the percentage consuming diet drinks was higher among females compared with males. The percentage consuming diet drinks was similar for females and males at all ages except among 12- to 19-year-olds, where a higher percentage of females than males consumed diet drinks. A higher percentage of non-Hispanic white persons consumed diet drinks compared with non-Hispanic black and Hispanic persons. The study included calorie-free and low-calorie versions of soft drinks, fruit drinks, energy drinks, sports drinks, and carbonated water.

ACES

Antioxidant supplements with varying amounts of carotene(s) for (pro) vitamin A, vitamin C, vitamin E and Selenium are known by the acronym, ACES. The commercial ACES formulas are a first generation, high potency, combined antioxidant that vary in component concentrations, specific components or source, and their ratio according to manufacturer and are available as both tablet and capsule. Vitamin supplementation will help those suffering from malnutrition, which in healthy individuals can be harmful, still obtaining the nutrients from fruit and vegetables instead is recommended, as supplementation is not proven to have any effectiveness in reducing occurrence of chronic disease.

Popularly known as "ACES" in the 1980s during a period of rapid commercial growth and public awareness, these formulas have frequently expanded and differentiated by adding minor amounts other antioxidants such as lipoic acid, pycnogenol, coenzyme Q-10, N-acetyl cysteine, as well as other nutrients that again vary with manufacturer, and are often simply referred to as super antioxidants or a branded, proprietary trade name.

Beta-carotene, one of over 600 carotenoids, has been the most common ingredient for vitamin A activity in ACES formulas. Ascorbic acid and ascorbates are the common ingredients to deliver vitamin C activity. Vitamin E content has commonly varied among d,l-alpha-tocopheryl acetate (all-rac alpha-tocopheryl acetate), d-alpha-tocopheryl acetate, d-alpha-tocopheryl succinate, and d-alpha-tocopherol. Selenium content has been delivered as selenate, selenium containing nutritional yeast and selenium containing organic forms such as L-Selenomethionine and L-selenium-methylselenocysteine, again varying with manufacturer. More recent ACES formulas may use mixed natural carotene sources that include other carotenes such as zeaxanthin, alpha carotene, cryptoxanthin, lutein and lycopene. Mixed tocopherols with varied proportions of R,R,R-alpha-tocopherol, R,R,R-beta-tocopherol, R,R,R-gamma-tocopherol and R,R,R-delta-tocopherol are other suitable sources of vitamin E content in ACES formulas.

Various ACES formulations will typically contain 10,000–25,000 IU carotenes, 250 mg – 1000 mg vitamin C, 200–400 IU alpha-tocopherol, and 50–200 µg selenium content per serving of one to three units (tablet or capsule), as well as other nutrients in more recent antioxidant formulations.

Vitamin A

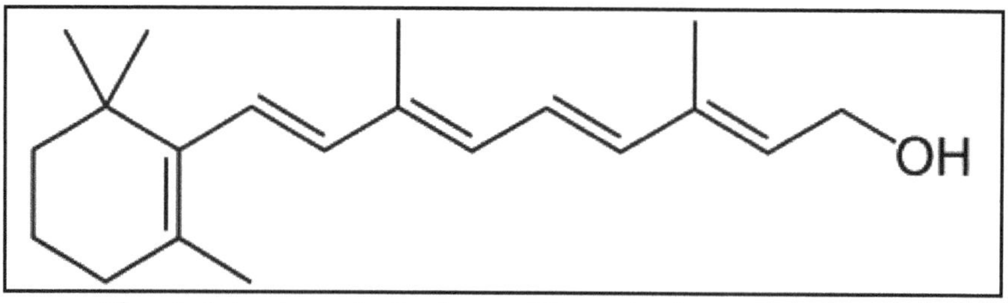

Chemical structure of retinol, one of the major forms of vitamin A.

Vitamin A is a group of unsaturated nutritional organic compounds that includes retinol, retinal, retinoic acid, and several provitamin A carotenoids (most notably beta-carotene). Vitamin A has multiple functions: it is important for growth and development, for the maintenance of the immune system and good vision. Vitamin A is needed by the retina of the eye in the form of retinal, which combines with protein opsin to form rhodopsin, the light-absorbing molecule necessary for both low-light (scotopic vision) and color vision. Vitamin A also functions in a very different role as retinoic acid (an irreversibly oxidized form of retinol), which is an important hormone-like growth factor for epithelial and other cells.

In foods of animal origin, the major form of vitamin A is an ester, primarily retinyl palmitate, which is converted to retinol (chemically an alcohol) in the small intestine. The retinol form functions as a storage form of the vitamin, and can be converted to and from its visually active aldehyde form, retinal.

All forms of vitamin A have a beta-ionone ring to which an isoprenoid chain is attached, called a *retinyl group*. Both structural features are essential for vitamin activity. The orange pigment of carrots (beta-carotene) can be represented as two connected retinyl groups, which are used in the body to contribute to vitamin A levels. Alpha-carotene and gamma-carotene also have a single retinyl group, which give them some vitamin activity. None of the other carotenes have vitamin activity. The carotenoid beta-cryptoxanthin possesses an ionone group and has vitamin activity in humans.

Vitamin A can be found in two principal forms in foods:

- Retinol, the form of vitamin A absorbed when eating animal food sources, is a yellow, fat-soluble substance. Since the pure alcohol form is unstable, the vitamin is found in tissues in a form of retinyl ester. It is also commercially produced and administered as esters such as retinyl acetate or palmitate.
- The carotenes alpha-carotene, beta-carotene, gamma-carotene; and the xanthophyll beta-cryptoxanthin (all of which contain beta-ionone rings), but no other carotenoids, function as provitamin A in herbivores and omnivore animals, which possess the enzyme beta-carotene 15,15'-dioxygenase which cleaves

beta-carotene in the intestinal mucosa and converts it to retinol. In general, carnivores are poor converters of ionone-containing carotenoids, and pure carnivores such as cats and ferrets lack beta-carotene 15,15'-dioxygenase and cannot convert any carotenoids to retinal (resulting in *none* of the carotenoids being forms of vitamin A for these species).

History

The discovery of vitamin A may have stemmed from research dating back to 1816, when physiologist François Magendie observed that dogs deprived of nutrition developed corneal ulcers and had a high mortality rate. In 1912, Frederick Gowland Hopkins demonstrated that unknown accessory factors found in milk, other than carbohydrates, proteins, and fats were necessary for growth in rats. Hopkins received a Nobel Prize for this discovery in 1929. By 1913, one of these substances was independently discovered by Elmer McCollum and Marguerite Davis at the University of Wisconsin–Madison, and Lafayette Mendel and Thomas Burr Osborne at Yale University who studied the role of fats in the diet. McCollum and Davis ultimately received credit because they submitted their paper three weeks before Mendel and Osborne. Both papers appeared in the same issue of the *Journal of Biological Chemistry* in 1913. The "accessory factors" were termed "fat soluble" in 1918 and later "vitamin A" in 1920. In 1919, Harry Steenbock (University of Wisconsin–Madison) proposed a relationship between yellow plant pigments (beta-carotene) and vitamin A. In 1931, Swiss chemist Paul Karrer described the chemical structure of vitamin A. Vitamin A was first synthesized in 1947 by two Dutch chemists, David Adriaan van Dorp and Jozef Ferdinand Arens.

Equivalencies of Retinoids and Carotenoids (IU)

As some carotenoids can be converted into vitamin A, attempts have been made to determine how much of them in the diet is equivalent to a particular amount of retinol, so that comparisons can be made of the benefit of different foods. The situation can be confusing because the accepted equivalences have changed. For many years, a system of equivalencies in which an international unit (IU) was equal to 0.3 μg of retinol, 0.6 μg of β-carotene, or 1.2 μg of other provitamin-A carotenoids was used. Later, a unit called retinol equivalent (RE) was introduced. Prior to 2001, one RE corresponded to 1 μg retinol, 2 μg β-carotene dissolved in oil (it is only partly dissolved in most supplement pills, due to very poor solubility in any medium), 6 μg β-carotene in normal food (because it is not absorbed as well as when in oils), and 12 μg of either α-carotene, γ-carotene, or β-cryptoxanthin in food.

Newer research has shown that the absorption of provitamin-A carotenoids is only half as much as previously thought. As a result, in 2001 the US Institute of Medicine recommended a new unit, the retinol activity equivalent (RAE). Each μg RAE corresponds to 1 μg retinol, 2 μg of β-carotene in oil, 12 μg of "dietary" beta-carotene, or 24 μg of the three other dietary provitamin-A carotenoids.

Substance and its chemical environment	Micrograms of retinol equivalent per microgram of the substance
retinol	1
beta-carotene, dissolved in oil	1/2
beta-carotene, common dietary	1/12
alpha-carotene, common dietary	1/24
gamma-carotene, common dietary	1/24
beta-cryptoxanthin, common dietary	1/24

Because the conversion of retinol from provitamin carotenoids by the human body is actively regulated by the amount of retinol available to the body, the conversions apply strictly only for vitamin A-deficient humans. The absorption of provitamins depends greatly on the amount of lipids ingested with the provitamin; lipids increase the uptake of the provitamin.

The conclusion that can be drawn from the newer research is that fruits and vegetables are not as useful for obtaining vitamin A as was thought; in other words, the IUs that these foods were reported to contain were worth much less than the same number of IUs of fat-dissolved oils and (to some extent) supplements. This is important for vegetarians, as night blindness is prevalent in countries where little meat or vitamin A-fortified foods are available.

A sample vegan diet for one day that provides sufficient vitamin A has been published by the Food and Nutrition Board (page 120). On the other hand, reference values for retinol or its equivalents, provided by the National Academy of Sciences, have decreased. The RDA (for men) of 1968 was 5000 IU (1500 μg retinol). In 1974, the RDA was set to 1000 RE (1000 μg retinol), whereas now the Dietary Reference Intake is 900 RAE (900 μg or 3000 IU retinol). This is equivalent to 1800 μg of β-carotene supplement (3000 IU) or 10800 μg of β-carotene in food (18000 IU).

Recommended Daily Allowance

Vitamin A

Dietary Reference Intake:

Life stage group	RDA Adequate intakes (AI*) μg/day	Upper limit μg/day
Infants		
0–6 months	400*	600
7–12 months	500*	600
Children		
1–3 years	300	600
4–8 years	400	900

Males 9–13 years 14–18 years 19 – >70 years	600 900 900	1700 2800 3000
Females 9–13 years 14–18 years 19 – >70 years	600 700 700	1700 2800 3000
Pregnancy <19 years 19 – >50 years	750 770	2800 3000
Lactation <19 years 19 – >50 years	1200 1300	2800 3000

(The limit is for synthetic and natural retinol ester forms of vitamin A. Carotene forms from dietary sources are not toxic.)

According to the Institute of Medicine of the National Academies, "RDAs are set to meet the needs of almost all (97 to 98%) individuals in a group. For healthy breastfed infants, the AI is the mean intake. The AI for other life stage and gender groups is believed to cover the needs of all individuals in the group, but lack of data prevents being able to specify with confidence the percentage of individuals covered by this intake."

Sources

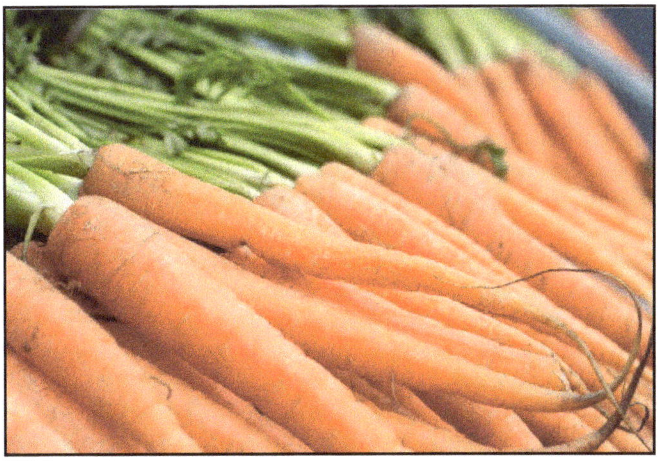

carrots

Vitamin A is found in many foods:

- cod liver oil (30000 μg 3333%).
- liver (turkey) (8058 μg 895%).

- liver (beef, pork, fish) (6500 µg 722%).
- liver (chicken) (3296 µg 366%).
- capsicum, red (2081 µg 231%).
- sweet potato (961 µg 107%).
- carrot (835 µg 93%).
- broccoli leaf (800 µg 89%).
- butter (684 µg 76%).
- kale (681 µg 76%).
- collard greens (frozen then boiled) (575 µg 64%).
- dandelion greens (508 µg 56%).
- spinach (469 µg 52%).
- pumpkin (426 µg 43%).
- collard greens (333 µg 37%).
- cheddar cheese (265 µg 29%).
- cantaloupe melon (169 µg 19%).
- egg (140 µg 16%).
- apricot (96 µg 11%).
- papaya (55 µg 6%).
- tomatoes (42 µg 5%).
- mango (38 µg 4%).
- pea (38 µg 4%).
- broccoli florets (31 µg 3%).
- milk (28 µg 3%).
- bell pepper, green (18 µg 2%).
- spirulina (3 µg 0.3%).

Note: Data taken from USDA database. Bracketed values are retinol activity equivalences (RAEs) and percentage of the adult male RDA, per 100 grams of the foodstuff (average).

Conversion of carotene to retinol varies from person to person and bioavailability of carotene in food varies.

Metabolic Functions

Vitamin A plays a role in a variety of functions throughout the body, such as:

- Vision.
- Gene transcription.
- Immune function.
- Embryonic development and reproduction.
- Bone metabolism.
- Haematopoiesis.
- Skin and cellular health.
- Antioxidant activity.

Vision

The role of vitamin A in the visual cycle is specifically related to the retinal form. Within the eye, 11-*cis*-retinal is bound to the protein "opsin" to form rhodopsin in rods and iodopsin (cones) at conserved lysine residues. As light enters the eye, the 11-*cis*-retinal is isomerized to the all-"trans" form. The all-"trans" retinal dissociates from the opsin in a series of steps called photo-bleaching. This isomerization induces a nervous signal along the optic nerve to the visual center of the brain. After separating from opsin, the all-"trans"-retinal is recycled and converted back to the 11-"cis"-retinal form by a series of enzymatic reactions. In addition, some of the all-"trans" retinal may be converted to all-"trans" retinol form and then transported with an interphotoreceptor retinol-binding protein (IRBP) to the pigment epithelial cells. Further esterification into all-"trans" retinyl esters allow for storage of all-trans-retinol within the pigment epithelial cells to be reused when needed. The final stage is conversion of 11-*cis*-retinal will rebind to opsin to reform rhodopsin (visual purple) in the retina. Rhodopsin is needed to see in low light (contrast) as well as for night vision. Kühne showed that rhodopsin in the retina is only regenerated when the retina is attached to retinal pigmented epithelium, which provides retinal. It is for this reason that a deficiency in vitamin A will inhibit the reformation of rhodopsin and lead to one of the first symptoms, night blindness.

Gene Transcription

Vitamin A, in the retinoic acid form, plays an important role in gene transcription. Once retinol has been taken up by a cell, it can be oxidized to retinal (retinaldehyde) by retinol dehydrogenases and then retinaldehyde can be oxidized to retinoic acid by retinaldehyde dehydrogenases. The conversion of retinaldehyde to retinoic acid is an irreversible step, meaning that the production of retinoic acid is tightly regulated, due to its activity as a ligand for nuclear receptors. The physiological form of retinoic acid (all-trans-retinoic acid) regulates gene transcription by binding to nuclear receptors known as retinoic acid receptors (RARs) which are bound to DNA as heterodimers with retinoid "X" receptors (RXRs). RAR and RXR must dimerize before they can bind to the DNA. RAR will form a heterodimer with RXR (RAR-RXR), but it does not readily form a homodimer (RAR-RAR). RXR, on the other hand, may form a homodimer (RXR-RXR) and will form heterodimers with many other nuclear receptors as well, including the thyroid hormone receptor (RXR-TR), the Vitamin D_3 receptor (RXR-VDR), the peroxisome proliferator-activated receptor (RXR-PPAR) and the liver "X" receptor (RXR-LXR). The RAR-RXR heterodimer recognizes retinoic acid response elements (RAREs) on the DNA whereas the RXR-RXR homodimer recognizes retinoid "X" response elements (RXREs) on the DNA; although several RAREs near target genes have been shown to control physiological processes, this has not been demonstrated for RXREs. The heterodimers of RXR with nuclear receptors other than RAR (i.e. TR, VDR, PPAR, LXR) bind to various distinct response elements on the DNA to control processes not regulated by vitamin A. Upon binding of retinoic acid to the RAR component of the RAR-RXR heterodimer, the receptors undergo a conformational change that causes co-repressors to dissociate from the receptors. Coactivators can then bind to the receptor complex, which may help to loosen the chromatin structure from the histones or may interact with the transcriptional machinery. This response can upregulate (or downregulate) the expression of target genes, including Hox genes as well as the genes that encode for the receptors themselves (i.e. RAR-beta in mammals).

Dermatology

Vitamin A, and more specifically, retinoic acid, appears to maintain normal skin health by switching on genes and differentiating keratinocytes (immature skin cells) into mature epidermal cells. Exact mechanisms behind pharmacological retinoid therapy agents in the treatment of dermatological diseases are being researched. For the treatment of acne, the most prescribed retinoid drug is 13-cis retinoic acid (isotretinoin). It reduces the size and secretion of the sebaceous glands. Although it is known that 40 mg of isotretinoin will break down to an equivalent of 10 mg of ATRA – the mechanism of action of the drug (original brand name Accutane) remains unknown and is a matter of some controversy. Isotretinoin reduces bacterial numbers in both the ducts and skin surface. This is thought to be a result of the reduction in sebum, a nutrient source for the bacteria. Isotretinoin reduces inflammation via inhibition of chemotactic responses of monocytes and neutrophils. Isotretinoin also has been shown to initiate remodeling of the sebaceous glands; triggering changes in gene expression that selectively induce apoptosis. Isotretinoin is a teratogen with a number of potential side-effects. Consequently, its use requires medical supervision.

Retinal/Retinol Versus Retinoic Acid

Vitamin A deprived rats can be kept in good general health with supplementation of retinoic acid. This reverses the growth-stunting effects of vitamin A deficiency, as well as early stages of xerophthalmia. However, such rats show infertility (in both male and females) and continued degeneration of the retina, showing that these functions require retinal or retinol, which are interconvertible but which cannot be recovered from the oxidized retinoic acid. The requirement of retinol to rescue reproduction in vitamin A deficient rats is now known to be due to a requirement for local synthesis of retinoic acid from retinol in testis and embryos.

Deficiency

Vitamin A deficiency is estimated to affect approximately one third of children under the age of five around the world. It is estimated to claim the lives of 670,000 children under five annually. Approximately 250,000–500,000 children in developing countries become blind each year owing to vitamin A deficiency, with the highest prevalence in Southeast Asia and Africa. Vitamin A deficiency is "the leading cause of preventable childhood blindness," according to UNICEF. It also increases the risk of death from common childhood conditions such as diarrhea. UNICEF regards addressing vitamin A deficiency as critical to reducing child mortality, the fourth of the United Nations' Millennium Development Goals.

Vitamin A deficiency can occur as either a primary or a secondary deficiency. A primary vitamin A deficiency occurs among children and adults who do not consume an adequate intake of provitamin A carotenoids from fruits and vegetables or preformed vitamin A from animal and dairy products. Early weaning from breastmilk can also increase the risk of vitamin A deficiency.

Secondary vitamin A deficiency is associated with chronic malabsorption of lipids, impaired bile production and release, and chronic exposure to oxidants, such as cigarette smoke, and chronic alcoholism. Vitamin A is a fat-soluble vitamin and depends on micellar solubilization for dispersion into the small intestine, which results in poor use of vitamin A from low-fat diets. Zinc deficiency can also impair absorption, transport, and metabolism of vitamin A because it is essential for the synthesis of the vitamin A transport proteins and as the cofactor in conversion of retinol to retinal. In malnourished populations, common low intakes of vitamin A and zinc increase the severity of vitamin A deficiency and lead physiological signs and symptoms of deficiency. A study in Burkina Faso showed major reduction of malaria morbidity with combined vitamin A and zinc supplementation in young children.

Due to the unique function of retinal as a visual chromophore, one of the earliest and specific manifestations of vitamin A deficiency is impaired vision, particularly in reduced light – night blindness. Persistent deficiency gives rise to a series of changes, the most devastating of which occur in the eyes. Some other ocular changes are referred to as xerophthalmia. First there is dryness of the conjunctiva (xerosis) as the normal lacrimal and mucus-secreting epithelium is replaced by a keratinized epithelium. This is followed by the build-up of keratin debris in small opaque plaques (Bitot's spots) and, eventually, erosion of the roughened corneal surface with softening and destruction of the cornea (keratomalacia) and leading to total blindness. Other changes include impaired immunity (increased risk of ear infections, urinary tract infections, Meningococcal disease), hyperkeratosis (white lumps at hair follicles), keratosis pilaris and squamous metaplasia of the epithelium lining the upper respiratory passages and urinary bladder to a keratinized epithelium. With relations to dentistry, a deficiency in Vitamin A leads to enamel hypoplasia.

Adequate supply, but not excess vitamin A, is especially important for pregnant and breastfeeding women for normal fetal development and in breastmilk. Deficiencies cannot be compensated by postnatal supplementation. Excess vitamin A, which is most common with high dose vitamin supplements, can cause birth defects and therefore should not exceed recommended daily values.

Vitamin A metabolic inhibition as a result of alcohol consumption during pregnancy is the elucidated mechanism for fetal alcohol syndrome and is characterized by teratogenicity closely matching maternal vitamin A deficiency.

Vitamin A Supplementation

Global efforts to support national governments in addressing vitamin A deficiency are led by the Global Alliance for Vitamin A (GAVA), which is an informal partnership between A2Z, the Canadian International Development Agency, Helen Keller International, the Micronutrient Initiative, UNICEF, USAID, and the World Bank. Joint GAVA activity is coordinated by the Micronutrient Initiative.

While strategies include intake of vitamin A through a combination of breast feeding and dietary intake, delivery of oral high-dose supplements remain the principal strategy for minimizing deficiency. A meta-analysis of 43 studies showed that vitamin A supplementation of children under five who are at risk of deficiency reduces mortality by up to 24%. About 75% of the vitamin A required for supplementation activity by developing countries is supplied by the Micronutrient Initiative with support from the Canadian International Development Agency. Food fortification approaches are becoming increasingly feasible but cannot yet ensure coverage levels.

The World Health Organization estimates that Vitamin A supplementation has averted 1.25 million deaths due to vitamin A deficiency in 40 countries since 1998. In 2008 it was estimated that an annual investment of US$60 million in vitamin A and zinc supplementation combined would yield benefits of more than US$1 billion per year, with every dollar spent generating benefits of more than US$17. These combined interventions were ranked by the Copenhagen Consensus 2008 as the world's best development investment.

Observational studies of pregnant women in sub-Saharan Africa have shown that low serum vitamin A levels are associated with an increased risk of mother-to-child transmission (MTCT) of HIV. Vitamin A is cheap and easily provided through existing health services in low-income settings. It is thus important to determine the effect of routine supplementation of H levels, and because low blood vitamin A levels have been associated with rapid HIV infection and deaths, To identify randomised controlled trials comparing vitamin A supplementation with placebo in known HIV-infected pregnant women, authors searched the Cochrane Library, PubMed, EMBASE, AIDSearch and GATEWAY; checked reference lis,. Authoritative reviews of more recent and better-designed studies have found no relationship between the level of serum maternal and/ or infant vitamin A and the likelihood of vertical (MTCT) HIV transmission. of HIV, our trials which enrolled 3033 HIV-infected pregnant women met inclusion criteria. Authors found significant statistical heterogeneity between the three trials with information on MTCT of HIV. Overall, there was no evidence of an effect of antenatal vitamin A supplementation on the risk of MTCT of HIV. However, antenatal vitamin A supplementation significantly improved birth weight, but there was no evidence of an effect on preterm births, stillbirths, deaths by 24 months.

Toxicity

Since vitamin A is fat-soluble, disposing of any excesses taken in through diet takes much longer than with water-soluble B vitamins and vitamin C. This allows for toxic levels of vitamin A to accumulate. These toxicities only occur with preformed (retinoid) vitamin A (such as from liver). The carotenoid forms (such as beta-carotene as found in carrots), give no such symptoms, except with supplements and chronic alcoholism, but excessive dietary intake of beta-carotene can lead to carotenodermia, a harmless but cosmetically displeasing orange-yellow discoloration of the skin.

In general, acute toxicity occurs at doses of 25,000 IU/kg of body weight, with chronic toxicity occurring at 4,000 IU/kg of body weight daily for 6–15 months. However, liver toxicities can occur at levels as low as 15,000 IU (4500 micrograms) per day to 1.4 million IU per day, with an average daily toxic dose of 120,000 IU, particularly with excessive consumption of alcohol . In people with renal failure, 4000 IU can cause substantial damage. Children can reach toxic levels at 1,500 IU/kg of body weight.

Excessive vitamin A consumption can lead to nausea, irritability, anorexia (reduced appetite), vomiting, blurry vision, headaches, hair loss, muscle and abdominal pain and weakness, drowsiness, and altered mental status. In chronic cases, hair loss, dry skin, drying of the mucous membranes, fever, insomnia, fatigue, weight loss, bone fractures, anemia, and diarrhea can all be evident on top of the symptoms associated with less serious toxicity. Some of these symptoms are also common to acne treatment with Isotretinoin. Chronically high doses of vitamin A, and also pharmaceutical retinoids such as 13-cis retinoic acid, can produce the syndrome of pseudotumor cerebri. This syndrome includes headache, blurring of vision and confusion, associated with increased intracerebral pressure. Symptoms begin to resolve when intake of the offending substance is stopped.

Chronic intake of 1500 RAE of preformed vitamin A may be associated with osteoporosis and hip fractures because it suppresses bone building while simultaneously stimulating bone breakdown.

High vitamin A intake has been associated with spontaneous bone fractures in animals. Cell culture studies have linked increased bone resorption and decreased bone formation with high intakes. This interaction may occur because vitamins A and D may compete for the same receptor and then interact with parathyroid hormone, which regulates calcium. Indeed, a study by Forsmo *et al.* shows a correlation between low bone mineral density and too high intake of vitamin A. Sufficiently high levels of vitamin D may be protective against the bone density lowering effects of high vitamin A, while inadequate levels of vitamin D may exacerbate those effects.

Toxic effects of vitamin A have been shown to significantly affect developing fetuses. Therapeutic doses used for acne treatment have been shown to disrupt cephalic neural cell activity. The fetus is particularly sensitive to vitamin A toxicity during the period of organogenesis.

Hepatic (liver) injury has been found in human and animal studies where consumption of alcohol is paired with high dose vitamin A and beta-carotene supplementation.

Researchers have succeeded in creating water-soluble forms of vitamin A, which they believed could reduce the potential for toxicity. However, a 2003 study found water-soluble vitamin A was approximately 10 times as toxic as fat-soluble vitamin. A 2006 study found children given water-soluble vitamin A and D, which are typically fat-soluble, suffer from asthma twice as much as a control group supplemented with the fat-soluble vitamins.

In some studies, the use of Vitamin A supplements has been linked to an increased rate of mortality, but there is minimal evidence to show this.

Vitamin A and Derivatives in Medical Use

Retinyl palmitate has been used in skin creams, where it is broken down to retinol and ostensibly metabolised to retinoic acid, which has potent biological activity, as described above.

The retinoids (for example, 13-cis-retinoic acid) constitute a class of chemical compounds chemically related to retinoic acid, and are used in medicine to modulate gene functions in place of this compound. Like retinoic acid, the related compounds do not have full vitamin A activity, but do have powerful effects on gene expression and epithelial cell differentiation.

Pharmaceutics utilizing mega doses of naturally occurring retinoic acid derivatives are currently in use for cancer, HIV, and dermatological purposes. At high doses, side-effects are similar to vitamin A toxicity.

Vitamin C

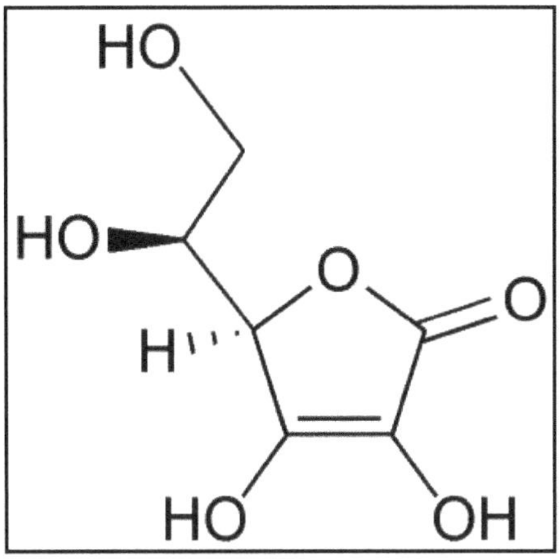

ascorbic acid
(reduced form).

Vitamin C is a cofactor in at least eight enzymatic reactions, including several collagen synthesis reactions that, when dysfunctional, cause the most severe symptoms of scurvy. In animals, these reactions are especially important in wound-healing and in preventing bleeding from capillaries. Ascorbate also acts as an antioxidant, protecting against oxidative stress.

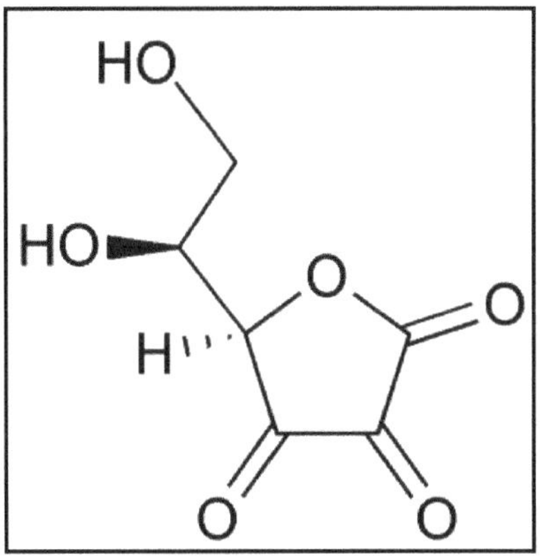

dehydroascorbic acid
(oxidized form).

Ascorbate (the anion of ascorbic acid) is required for a range of essential metabolic reactions in all animals and plants. It is made internally by almost all organisms; the main exceptions are most bats, all guinea pigs, capybaras, and the Haplorrhini (one of the two major primate suborders, consisting of tarsiers, monkeys, and humans and other apes). Ascorbate is also not synthesized by many species of birds and fish. All species that do not synthesize ascorbate require it in the diet. Deficiency in this vitamin causes the disease scurvy in humans.

Ascorbic acid is also widely used as a food additive, to prevent oxidation.

Vitamers

The name 'vitamin C' always refers to the L-enantiomer of ascorbic acid and its oxidized forms. The opposite D-enantiomer called D-ascorbate has equal antioxidant power, but is not found in nature, and has no physiological significance. When D-ascorbate is synthesized and given to animals that require vitamin C in their diets, it has been found to have far less vitamin activity than the L-enantiomer. Therefore, unless written otherwise, "ascorbate" and "ascorbic acid" refer in the nutritional literature to L-ascorbate and L-ascorbic acid, respectively. This notation will be followed in this article. Similarly, their oxidized derivatives are all L-enantiomers, and also need not be written with full stereochemical notation here.

Ascorbic acid is a weak sugar acid structurally related to glucose. In biological systems, ascorbic acid can be found only at low pH, but in neutral solutions above pH 5 is predominantly found in the ionized form, ascorbate. All of these molecules have vitamin C activity, therefore, and are used synonymously with vitamin C, unless otherwise specified.

Biological Significance

The biological role of ascorbate is to act as a reducing agent, donating electrons to various enzymatic and a few non-enzymatic reactions. The one- and two-electron oxidized forms of vitamin C, semidehydroascorbic acid and dehydroascorbic acid, respectively, can be reduced in the body by glutathione and NADPH-dependent enzymatic mechanisms. The presence of glutathione in cells and extracellular fluids helps maintain ascorbate in a reduced state.

Biosynthesis

The vast majority of animals and plants are able to synthesize vitamin C, through a sequence of enzyme-driven steps, which convert monosaccharides to vitamin C. In plants, this is accomplished through the conversion of mannose or galactose to ascorbic acid. In some animals, glucose needed to produce ascorbate in the liver (in mammals and perching birds) is extracted from glycogen; ascorbate synthesis is a glycogenolysis-dependent process. In reptiles and birds the biosynthesis is carried out in the kidneys.

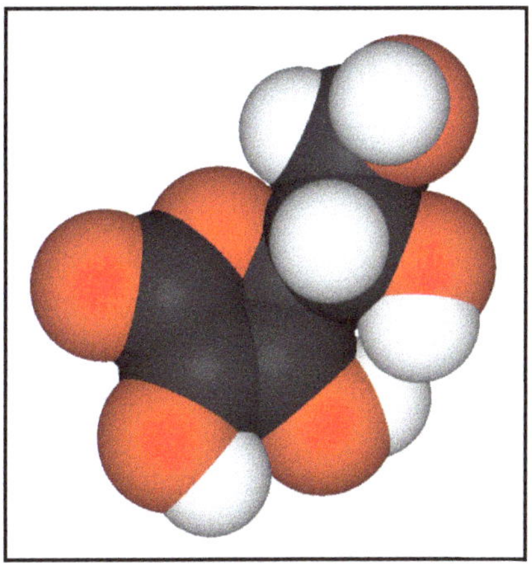

Model of a vitamin C molecule. Black is carbon, red is oxygen, and white is hydrogen.

Among the animals that have lost the ability to synthesize vitamin C are simians and tarsiers, which together make up one of two major primate suborders, Haplorrhini. This group includes humans. The other more primitive primates (Strepsirrhini) have the ability to make vitamin C. Synthesis does not occur in a number of species (perhaps all species) in the small rodent family Caviidae that includes guinea pigs and capybaras, but occurs in other rodents (rats and mice do not need vitamin C in their diet, for example).

A number of species of passerine birds also do not synthesize, but not all of them, and those that do not are not clearly related; there is a theory that the ability was lost separately a number of times in birds. In particular, the ability to synthesize vitamin C is presumed to have been lost and then later re-acquired in at least two cases.

All tested families of bats (Order Chiroptera), including major insect and fruit-eating bat families, cannot synthesize vitamin C. A trace of gulonolactone oxidase (GULO) was detected in only 1 of 34 bat species tested, across the range of 6 families of bats tested. However, recent results show that there are at least two species of bats, frugivorous bat (*Rousettus leschenaultii*) and insectivorous bat (*Hipposideros armiger*), that retain their ability of vitamin C production. The ability to synthesize vitamin C has also been lost in about 96% of fish (the teleosts).

These animals all lack the L-gulonolactone oxidase (GULO) enzyme, which is required in the last step of vitamin C synthesis, because they have a differing non-synthesizing gene for the enzyme (Pseudogene ΨGULO). A similar non-functional gene is present in the genome of the guinea pigs and in primates, including humans. Some of these species (including humans) are able to make do with the lower levels available from their diets by recycling oxidised vitamin C.

Most simians consume the vitamin in amounts 10 to 20 times higher than that recommended by governments for humans. This discrepancy constitutes much of the basis of the controversy on current recommended dietary allowances. It is countered by arguments that humans are very good at conserving dietary vitamin C, and are able to maintain blood levels of vitamin C comparable with other simians, on a far smaller dietary intake.

Like plants and animals, some microorganisms such as the yeast *Saccharomyces cerevisiae* have been shown to be able to synthesize vitamin C from simple sugars.

Evolution

Ascorbic acid or vitamin C is a common enzymatic cofactor in mammals used in the synthesis of collagen. Ascorbate is a powerful reducing agent capable of rapidly scavenging a number of reactive oxygen species (ROS). Freshwater teleost fishes also require dietary vitamin C in their diet or they will get scurvy. The most widely recognized symptoms of vitamin C deficiency in fishes are scoliosis, lordosis and dark skin coloration. Freshwater salmonids also show impaired collagen formation, internal/fin hemorrhage, spinal curvature and increased mortality. If these fishes are housed in seawater with algae and phytoplankton, then vitamin supplementation seems to be less important, it is presumed because of the availability of other, more ancient, antioxidants in natural marine environment.

Some scientists have suggested that loss of the vitamin C biosynthesis pathway may have played a role in rapid evolutionary changes, leading to hominids and the emergence of human beings. However, another theory is that the loss of ability to make vitamin C in simians may have occurred much farther back in evolutionary history than the emergence of humans or even apes, since it evidently occurred soon after the appearance of the first primates, yet sometime after the split of early primates into the two major suborders Haplorrhini (which cannot make vitamin C) and its sister suborder of non-tarsier prosimians, the Strepsirrhini ("wet-nosed" primates), which retained the ability to make vitamin C. According to molecular clock dating, these two suborder primate branches parted ways about 63 to 60 Mya. Approximately three to five million years later (58 Mya), only a short time afterward from an evolutionary perspective, the infraorder Tarsiiformes, whose only remaining family is that of the tarsier (Tarsiidae), branched off from the other haplorrhines. Since tarsiers also cannot make vitamin C, this implies the mutation had already occurred, and thus must have occurred between these two marker points (63 to 58 Mya).

It has been noted that the loss of the ability to synthesize ascorbate strikingly parallels the inability to break down uric acid, also a characteristic of primates. Uric acid and ascorbate are both strong reducing agents. This has led to the suggestion that, in higher primates, uric acid has taken over some of the functions of ascorbate.

Absorption, Transport, and Excretion

Ascorbic acid is absorbed in the body by both active transport and simple diffusion. Sodium-Dependent Active Transport—Sodium-Ascorbate Co-Transporters (SVCTs) and

Hexose transporters (GLUTs)—are the two transporters required for absorption. SVCT1 and SVCT2 import the reduced form of ascorbate across plasma membrane. GLUT1 and GLUT3 are the two glucose transporters, and transfer only the dehydroascorbic acid form of Vitamin C. Although dehydroascorbic acid is absorbed in higher rate than ascorbate, the amount of dehydroascorbic acid found in plasma and tissues under normal conditions is low, as cells rapidly reduce dehydroascorbic acid to ascorbate. Thus, SVCTs appear to be the predominant system for vitamin C transport in the body.

SVCT2 is involved in vitamin C transport in almost every tissue, the notable exception being red blood cells, which lose SVCT proteins during maturation. "SVCT2 knockout" animals genetically engineered to lack this functional gene, die shortly after birth, suggesting that SVCT2-mediated vitamin C transport is necessary for life.

With regular intake the absorption rate varies between 70 and 95%. However, the degree of absorption decreases as intake increases. At high intake (1.25 g), fractional human absorption of ascorbic acid may be as low as 33%; at low intake (<200 mg) the absorption rate can reach up to 98%.

Ascorbate concentrations over the renal re-absorption threshold pass freely into the urine and are excreted. At high dietary doses (corresponding to several hundred mg/day in humans) ascorbate is accumulated in the body until the plasma levels reach the renal resorption threshold, which is about 1.5 mg/dL in men and 1.3 mg/dL in women. Concentrations in the plasma larger than this value (thought to represent body saturation) are rapidly excreted in the urine with a half-life of about 30 minutes. Concentrations less than this threshold amount are actively retained by the kidneys, and the excretion half-life for the remainder of the vitamin C store in the body thus increases greatly, with the half-life lengthening as the body stores are depleted. This half-life rises until it is as long as 83 days by the onset of the first symptoms of scurvy.

Although the body's maximal store of vitamin C is largely determined by the renal threshold for blood, there are many tissues that maintain vitamin C concentrations far higher than in blood. Biological tissues that accumulate over 100 times the level in blood plasma of vitamin C are the adrenal glands, pituitary, thymus, corpus luteum, and retina. Those with 10 to 50 times the concentration present in blood plasma include the brain, spleen, lung, testicle, lymph nodes, liver, thyroid, small intestinal mucosa, leukocytes, pancreas, kidney, and salivary glands.

Ascorbic acid can be oxidized (broken down) in the human body by the enzyme L-ascorbate oxidase. Ascorbate that is not directly excreted in the urine as a result of body saturation or destroyed in other body metabolism is oxidized by this enzyme and removed.

Deficiency

Scurvy is an avitaminosis resulting from lack of vitamin C, since without this vitamin, the synthesized collagen is too unstable to perform its function. Scurvy leads to the formation of brown spots on the skin, spongy gums, and bleeding from all mucous membranes. The spots are most abundant on the thighs and legs, and a person with the ailment looks pale, feels depressed, and is partially immobilized. In advanced scurvy there are open, suppurating wounds and loss of teeth and, eventually, death. The human body can store only a certain amount of vitamin C, and so the body stores are depleted if fresh supplies are not consumed. The time frame for onset of symptoms of scurvy in unstressed adults on a completely vitamin C free diet, however, may range from one month to more than six months, depending on previous loading of vitamin C.

Western societies generally consume far more than sufficient vitamin C to prevent scurvy. In 2004, a Canadian Community health survey reported that Canadians of 19 years and above have intakes of vitamin C from food of 133 mg/d for males and 120 mg/d for females; these are higher than the RDA recommendations.

Notable human dietary studies of experimentally induced scurvy have been conducted on conscientious objectors during WW II in Britain, and on Iowa state prisoners in the late 1960s to the 1980s. These studies both found that all obvious symptoms of scurvy previously induced by an experimental scorbutic diet with extremely low vitamin C content could be completely reversed by additional vitamin C supplementation of only 10 mg a day. In these experiments, there was no clinical difference noted between men given 70 mg vitamin C per day (which produced blood level of vitamin C of about 0.55 mg/dl, about 1/3 of tissue saturation levels), and those given 10 mg per day. Men in the prison study developed the first signs of scurvy about 4 weeks after starting the vitamin C free diet, whereas in the British study, six to eight months were required, possibly due to the pre-loading of this group with a 70 mg/day supplement for six weeks before the scorbutic diet was fed.

Men in both studies on a diet devoid, or nearly devoid, of vitamin C had blood levels of vitamin C too low to be accurately measured when they developed signs of scurvy, and in the Iowa study, at this time were estimated (by labeled vitamin C dilution) to have a body pool of less than 300 mg, with daily turnover of only 2.5 mg/day, implying an instantaneous half-life of 83 days by this time (elimination constant of 4 months).

Supplementation

Studies of the potential of vitamin C supplementation to provide health benefits have provided conflicting results.

A 2013 systematic review by the U.S. Preventative Diseases Task Force found no clear evidence that vitamin C supplementation conferred benefit in the prevention of cardiovascular disease or cancer.Similarly, a 2012 Cochrane review found no effect of vitamin C supplementation on overall mortality. A 2014 meta-analysis found weak evidence of vitamin C protection against lung cancer risk.

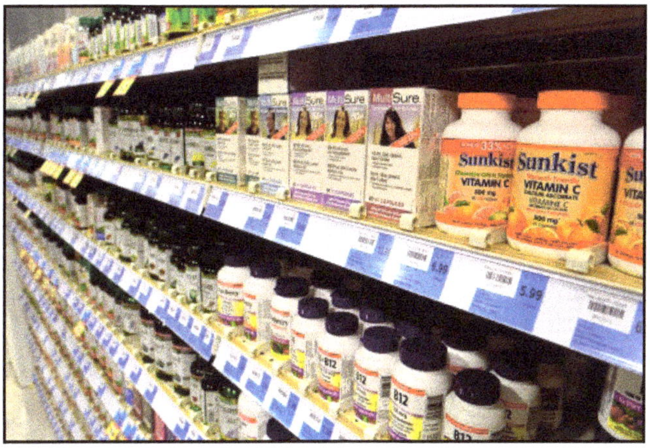

Vitamin C supplements at a drug store.

Cancer Prevention

A 2014 review found that, "Currently, the use of high-dose IV vitamin C [as an anticancer agent] cannot be recommended outside of a clinical trial."

A 2013 Cochrane review found no evidence that vitamin C supplementation reduces the risk of lung cancer in healthy or high risk (smokers and asbestos-exposed) people. A 2014 meta-analysis found weak evidence that vitamin C intake might protect against lung cancer risk. A second meta analysis found no effect on the risk of prostate cancer.

Two meta analyses evaluated the effect of vitamin C supplementation on the risk of colorectal cancer. One found a weak association between vitamin C consumption and reduced risk, and the other found no effect of supplementation.

A 2011 meta analysis failed to find support for the prevention of breast cancer with vitamin C supplementation, but a second study concluded that vitamin C may be associated with increased survival in those already diagnosed.

Cardiovascular Disease

A 2013 meta analysis found no evidence that vitamin C supplementation reduces the risk of myocardial infarction, stroke, cardiovascular mortality, or all-cause mortality. However, a second analysis found an inverse relationship between circulating vitamin C levels or dietary vitamin C and the risk of stroke.

A meta-analysis of 44 clinical trials has shown a significant positive effect of vitamin C on endothelial function when taken at doses greater than 500 mg per day. The researchers noted that the effect of vitamin C supplementation appeared to be dependent on health status, with stronger effects in those at higher cardiovascular disease risk.

Chronic Diseases

A 2010 review in the journal *Alternative Therapies in Health and Medicine* found no role for vitamin C supplementation in the treatment of rheumatoid arthritis.

Studies examining the effects of vitamin C intake on the risk of Alzheimer's disease have reached conflicting conclusions. Maintaining a healthy dietary intake is probably more important than supplementation for achieving any potential benefit.

Vitamin C supplementation above the RDA has been used in trials to study a potential effect on preventing and slowing the progression of age-related cataract, however no significant effects were found from the research.

Treatment of the Common Cold

Vitamin C's effect on the common cold has been extensively researched. It has not been shown effective in prevention or treatment of the common cold, except in limited circumstances (specifically, individuals exercising vigorously in cold environments). Routine vitamin C supplementation does not reduce the incidence or severity of the common cold in the general population, though it may reduce the duration of illness.

Role in Mammals

In humans, vitamin C is essential to a healthy diet as well as being a highly effective antioxidant, acting to lessen oxidative stress; a substrate for ascorbate peroxidase in plants (APX is plant specific enzyme); and an enzyme cofactor for the biosynthesis of many important biochemicals. Vitamin C acts as an electron donor for important enzymes:

Enzymatic Cofactor

Ascorbic acid performs numerous physiological functions in the human body. These functions include the synthesis of collagen, carnitine, and neurotransmitters; the synthesis and catabolism of tyrosine; and the metabolism of microsome. During biosynthesis ascorbate acts as a reducing agent, donating electrons and preventing oxidation to keep iron and copper atoms in their reduced states.

Vitamin C acts as an electron donor for eight different enzymes:

- Three enzymes (prolyl-3-hydroxylase, prolyl-4-hydroxylase, and lysyl hydroxylase) that are required for the hydroxylation of proline and lysine in the synthesis of collagen. These reactions add hydroxyl groups to the amino acids proline or lysine in the collagen molecule via prolyl hydroxylase and lysyl hydroxylase, both requiring vitamin C as a cofactor. Hydroxylation allows the collagen molecule to assume its triple helix structure, and thus vitamin C is essential to the development and maintenance of scar tissue, blood vessels, and cartilage.

- Two enzymes (ε-N-trimethyl-L-lysine hydroxylase and γ-butyrobetaine hydroxylase) that are necessary for synthesis of carnitine. Carnitine is essential for the transport of fatty acids into mitochondria for ATP generation.
- The remaining three enzymes have the following functions in common, but have other functions as well:
    - dopamine beta hydroxylase participates in the biosynthesis of norepinephrine from dopamine.
    - Peptidylglycine alpha-amidating monooxygenase amidates peptide hormones by removing the glyoxylate residue from their c-terminal glycine residues. This increases peptide hormone stability and activity.
    - 4-hydroxyphenylpyruvate dioxygenase modulates tyrosine metabolism.

Immune System

Vitamin C is found in high concentrations in immune cells, and is consumed quickly during infections. It is not certain how vitamin C interacts with the immune system; it has been hypothesized to modulate the activities of phagocytes, the production of cytokines and lymphocytes, and the number of cell adhesion molecules in monocytes.

Role in Plants

Ascorbic acid is associated with chloroplasts and apparently plays a role in ameliorating the oxidative stress of photosynthesis. In addition, it has a number of other roles in cell division and protein modification. Plants appear to be able to make ascorbate by at least one other biochemical route that is different from the major route in animals, although precise details remain unknown.

Daily Requirements

The North American Dietary Reference Intake recommends 90 milligrams per day for adult men, 75 mg/day for adult women, and no more than 2 grams (2,000 milligrams) per day. There is continuing debate within the scientific community over the best dose schedule (the amount and frequency of intake) of vitamin C for maintaining optimal health in humans. A 2008 review recommended 1,000 mg/day as a supplement, in addition to what is consumed from food. A balanced diet without supplementation usually contains enough vitamin C to prevent scurvy in an average healthy adult, while those who smoke tobacco or are under stress require slightly more.

United States vitamin C recommendations	
Recommended Dietary Allowance (adult male)	90 mg per day

Recommended Dietary Allowance (adult female)	75 mg per day
Recommended Dietary Allowance (pregnancy)	85 mg per day
Recommended Dietary Allowance (lactation)	120 mg per day
Tolerable Upper Intake Level (adult male)	2,000 mg per day
Tolerable Upper Intake Level (adult female)	2,000 mg per day

Government Recommended Intake

Recommendations for vitamin C intake have been set by various national agencies:

- 40 milligrams per day or 280 milligrams per week taken all at once: the United Kingdom's Food Standards Agency.
- 40 milligrams per day as per the recommendations of India's National Institute of Nutrition, Hyderabad.
- 45 milligrams per day 300 milligrams per week: the World Health Organization.
- 80 milligrams per day: the European Commission's Council on nutrition labeling.
- 90 mg/day (males) and 75 mg/day (females): Health Canada 2007.
- 90 mg/day (males) and 75 mg/day (females): United States' National Academy of Sciences.
- 100 milligrams per day: Japan's National Institute of Health and Nutrition.

For U.S. food and dietary supplement labeling purposes the amount in a serving is expressed as a percent of Daily Value (%DV). For vitamin C labeling purposes 100% of the Daily Value was 60 mg, but as of May 2016 it has been revised to 90 mg. A table of the pre-change adult Daily Values is provided at Reference Daily Intake. Food and supplement companies have until July 28, 2018 to comply with the change.

Testing for Ascorbate Levels in the Body

Simple tests use dichlorophenolindophenol, a redox indicator, to measure the levels of vitamin C in the urine and in serum or blood plasma. However these reflect recent dietary intake rather than the level of vitamin C in body stores. Reverse phase high performance liquid chromatography is used for determining the storage levels of vitamin C within lymphocytes and tissue. It has been observed that while serum or blood plasma levels follow the circadian rhythm or short term dietary changes, those within tissues themselves are more stable and give a better view of the availability of ascorbate within the organism. However, very few hospital laboratories are adequately equipped and trained to carry out such detailed analyses, and require samples to be analyzed in specialized laboratories.

Adverse Effects

Common Side-effects

Relatively large doses of ascorbic acid may cause indigestion, particularly when taken on an empty stomach. However, taking vitamin C in the form of sodium ascorbate and calcium ascorbate may minimize this effect. When taken in large doses, ascorbic acid causes diarrhea in healthy subjects. In one trial in 1936, doses of up to 6 grams of ascorbic acid were given to 29 infants, 93 children of preschool and school age, and 20 adults for more than 1400 days. With the higher doses, toxic manifestations were observed in five adults and four infants. The signs and symptoms in adults were nausea, vomiting, diarrhea, flushing of the face, headache, fatigue and disturbed sleep. The main toxic reactions in the infants were skin rashes.

Possible Side-effects

As vitamin C enhances iron absorption, iron poisoning can become an issue to people with rare iron overload disorders, such as haemochromatosis. A genetic condition that results in inadequate levels of the enzyme glucose-6-phosphate dehydrogenase (G6PD) can cause sufferers to develop hemolytic anemia after ingesting specific oxidizing substances, such as very large dosages of vitamin C.

There is a longstanding belief among the mainstream medical community that vitamin C causes kidney stones, which is based on little science. Although recent studies have found a relationship, a clear link between excess ascorbic acid intake and kidney stone formation has not been generally established. Some case reports exist for a link between patients with oxalate deposits and a history of high-dose vitamin C usage.

In a study conducted on rats, during the first month of pregnancy, high doses of vitamin C may suppress the production of progesterone from the corpus luteum. Progesterone, necessary for the maintenance of a pregnancy, is produced by the corpus luteum for the first few weeks, until the placenta is developed enough to produce its own source. By blocking this function of the corpus luteum, high doses of vitamin C (1000+ mg) are theorized to induce an early miscarriage. In a group of spontaneously aborting women at the end of the first trimester, the mean values of vitamin C were significantly higher in the aborting group. However, the authors do state: 'This could not be interpreted as an evidence of causal association.' However, in a previous study of 79 women with threatened, previous spontaneous, or habitual abortion, Javert and Stander (1943) had 91% success with 33 patients who received vitamin C together with bioflavonoids and vitamin K (only three abortions), whereas all of the 46 patients who did not receive the vitamins aborted.

A study in rats and humans suggested that adding Vitamin C supplements to an exercise training program lowered the expected effect of training on VO2 Max. Although the results in humans were not statistically significant, this study is often cited as evidence that high doses of Vitamin C have an adverse effect on exercise performance. In rats, it was shown that the additional Vitamin C resulted in lowered mitochondria production. Since rats are able to produce all of their needed Vitamin C, however, it is questionable whether they offer a relevant model of human physiological processes in this regard.

A cancer-causing mechanism of hexavalent chromium may be triggered by vitamin C.

Overdose

Vitamin C is water-soluble, with dietary excesses not absorbed, and excesses in the blood rapidly excreted in the urine. It exhibits remarkably low toxicity. The LD_{50} (the dose that will kill 50% of a population) in rats is generally accepted to be 11.9 grams per kilogram of body weight when given by forced gavage (orally). The mechanism of death from such doses (1.2% of body weight, or 0.84 kg for a 70 kg human) is unknown, but may be more mechanical than chemical. The LD_{50} in humans remains unknown, given lack of any accidental or intentional poisoning death data. However, as with all substances tested in this way, the rat LD_{50} is taken as a guide to its toxicity in humans.

In 2000 the Food and Nutrition Board of the National Academy of Sciences set a Tolerable Upper Intake Level (UL) of 2,000 mg/day. The amount was chosen because human trials had reported diarrhea and other gastrointestinal disturbances at intakes of greater than 3,000 mg/day. This was the Lowest-Observed-Adverse-Effect Level (LOAEL), meaning that other adverse effects were observed at higher intakes.

Dietary Sources

The richest natural sources are fruits and vegetables, and of those, the Kakadu plum and the camu camu fruit contain the highest concentration of the vitamin. It is also present in some cuts of meat, especially liver. Vitamin C is the most widely taken nutritional supplement and is available in a variety of forms, including tablets, drink mixes, crystals in capsules or naked crystals.

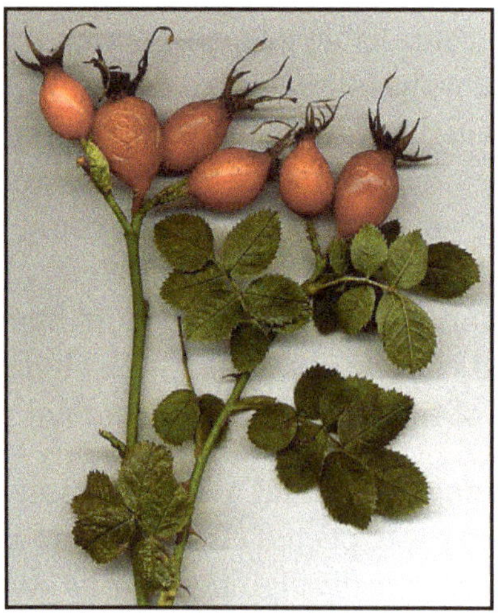

Rose hips are a particularly rich source of vitamin C.

Vitamin C is absorbed by the intestines using a sodium-ion dependent channel. It is transported through the intestine via both glucose-sensitive and glucose-insensitive mechanisms. The presence of large quantities of sugar either in the intestines or in the blood can slow absorption.

Plant Sources

While plants are generally a good source of vitamin C, the amount in foods of plant origin depends on the precise variety of the plant, soil condition, climate where it grew, length of time since it was picked, storage conditions, and method of preparation.

The following table is approximate and shows the relative abundance in different raw plant sources. As some plants were analyzed fresh while others were dried (thus, artifactually increasing concentration of individual constituents like vitamin C), the data are subject to potential variation and difficulties for comparison. The amount is given in milligrams per 100 grams of fruit or vegetable and is a rounded average from multiple authoritative sources:

Plant source	Amount (mg / 100g)
Kakadu plum	1000–5300
Camu Camu	2800
Acerola	1677
Seabuckthorn	695
Indian gooseberry	445
Rose hip	426
Baobab	400
Chili pepper (green)	244
Guava (common, raw)	228.3
Blackcurrant	200
Red pepper	190
Chili pepper (red)	144
Parsley	130
Kiwifruit	90
Broccoli	90
Loganberry	80
Redcurrant	80
Brussels sprouts	80
Wolfberry (Goji)	73 †
Lychee	70
Persimmon (native, raw)	66.0
Cloudberry	60
Elderberry	60

† average of 3 sources; dried

Plant source	Amount (mg / 100g)
Papaya	60
Strawberry	60
Orange	53
Lemon	53
Pineapple	48
Cauliflower	48
Kale	41
Melon, cantaloupe	40
Garlic	31
Grapefruit	30
Raspberry	30
Tangerine	30
Mandarin orange	30
Passion fruit	30
Spinach	30
Cabbage raw green	30
Lime	30
Mango	28
Rutabaga	25
Blackberry	21
Potato	20
Melon, honeydew	20
Tomato, red	13.7
Cranberry	13
Tomato	10
Blueberry	10
Pawpaw	10
Plant source	**Amount (mg / 100g)**
Grape	10
Apricot	10
Plum	10
Watermelon	10
Banana	9
Avocado	8.8
Crabapple	8

Onion	7.4
Cherry	7
Peach	7
Carrot	6
Apple	6
Asparagus	6
Horned melon	5.3
Beetroot	5
Chokecherry	5
Pear	4
Lettuce	4
Cucumber	3
Eggplant	2
Raisin	2
Fig	2
Bilberry	1
Medlar	0.3

Animal Sources

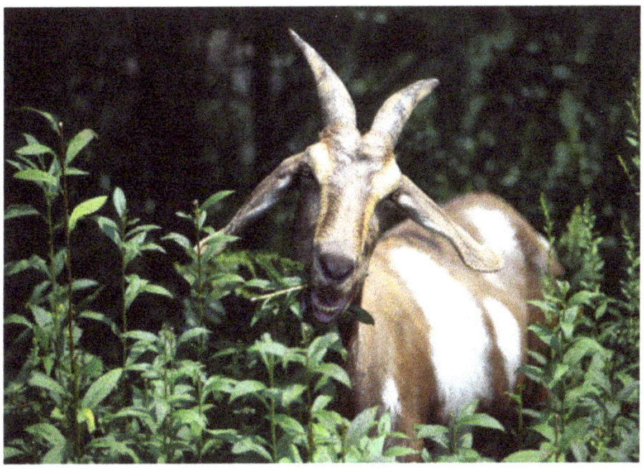

Goats, like almost all animals, make their own vitamin C. An adult goat, weighing approx. 70 kg, will manufacture more than 13,000 mg of vitamin C per day in normal health, and levels manyfold higher when faced with stress.

The overwhelming majority of species of animals (but *not* humans, guinea pigs or fruit bats) and plants synthesize their own vitamin C. Therefore, some animal products can be used as sources of dietary vitamin C.

Vitamin C is most present in the liver and least present in the muscle. Since muscle provides the majority of meat consumed in the western human diet, animal products are not a reliable source of the vitamin. Vitamin C is present in human breast milk, but only in limited quantity in raw cow's milk. All excess vitamin C is disposed of through the urinary system.

The following table shows the relative abundance of vitamin C in various foods of animal origin, given in milligrams of vitamin C per 100 grams of food:

Animal Source	Amount (mg / 100g)	
Calf liver (raw)	36	
Beef liver (raw)	31	
Oysters (raw)	30	
Cod roe (fried)	26	
Pork liver (raw)	23	
Lamb brain (boiled)	17	
Chicken liver (fried)	13	
Animal Source	**Amount (mg / 100g)**	
Lamb liver (fried)	12	
Calf adrenals (raw)	11	
Lamb heart (roast)	11	
Lamb tongue (stewed)	6	
Camel milk (fresh)	5	
Human milk (fresh)	4	
Goat milk (fresh)	2	
Cow milk (fresh)	2	

Food Preparation

Vitamin C chemically decomposes under certain conditions, many of which may occur during the cooking of food. Vitamin C concentrations in various food substances decrease with time in proportion to the temperature they are stored at and cooking can reduce the Vitamin C content of vegetables by around 60% possibly partly due to increased enzymatic destruction as it may be more significant at sub-boiling temperatures. Longer cooking times also add to this effect, as will copper food vessels, which catalyse the decomposition.

Another cause of vitamin C being lost from food is leaching, where the water-soluble vitamin dissolves into the cooking water, which is later poured away and not consumed. However, vitamin C does not leach in all vegetables at the same rate; research shows broccoli seems to retain more than any other. Research has also shown that freshly cut fruits do not lose significant nutrients when stored in the refrigerator for a few days.

Supplements

Vitamin C is available in caplets, tablets, capsules, drink mix packets, in multi-vitamin formulations, in multiple antioxidant formulations, and as crystalline powder. Timed release versions are available, as are formulations containing bioflavonoids such as quercetin, hesperidin, and rutin. Tablet and capsule sizes range from 25 mg to 1500 mg. Vitamin C (as ascorbic acid) crystals are typically available in bottles containing 300 g to 1 kg of powder (a 5 ml teaspoon of vitamin C crystals equals 5,000 mg). The bottles are usually airtight and brown or opaque in order to prevent oxidation, in which case the vitamin C would become useless, if not damaging.

Industrial Synthesis

Vitamin C is produced from glucose by two main routes. The Reichstein process, developed in the 1930s, uses a single pre-fermentation followed by a purely chemical route. The modern two-step fermentation process, originally developed in China in the 1960s, uses additional fermentation to replace part of the later chemical stages. Both processes yield approximately 60% vitamin C from the glucose feed.

Research is underway at the Scottish Crop Research Institute in the interest of creating a strain of yeast that can synthesize vitamin C in a single fermentation step from galactose, a technology expected to reduce manufacturing costs considerably.

World production of synthesized vitamin C is currently estimated at approximately 110,000 tonnes annually. The main producers have been BASF/Takeda, DSM, Merck and the China Pharmaceutical Group Ltd. of the People's Republic of China. By 2008 only the DSM plant in Scotland remained operational outside the strong price competition from China. The world price of vitamin C rose sharply in 2008 partly as a result of rises in basic food prices but also in anticipation of a stoppage of the two Chinese plants, situated at Shijiazhuang near Beijing, as part of a general shutdown of polluting industry in China over the period of the Olympic games. Five Chinese manufacturers met in 2010, among them Northeast Pharmaceutical Group and North China Pharmaceutical Group, and agreed to temporarily stop production in order to maintain prices. In 2011 an American suit was filed against four Chinese companies that allegedly colluded to limit production and fix prices of vitamin C in the United States. According to the plaintiffs, after the agreement was made spot prices for vitamin C shot to as high as $7 per kilogram in December 2002 from $2.50 per kilogram in December 2001. The companies did not deny the accusation but say in their defense that the Chinese government compelled them to act in this way. In January 2012 a US judge ruled that the Chinese companies can be sued in the U.S. by buyers acting as a group.

Food Fortification

In 2005, Health Canada evaluated the effect of fortification of foods with ascorbate in the guidance document, *Addition of Vitamins and Minerals to Food.* Ascorbate was categorized as a 'Risk Category A nutrient', meaning it is a nutrient for which an upper limit for intake is set but allows a wide margin of intake that has a narrow margin of safety but non-serious critical adverse effects.

Compendial Status

- British Pharmacopoeia.
- Japanese Pharmacopoeia.

History

James Lind, a British Royal Navy surgeon who, in 1747, identified that a quality in fruit prevented the disease of scurvy in what was the first recorded controlled experiment.

The need to include fresh plant food or raw animal flesh in the diet to prevent disease was known from ancient times. Native people living in marginal areas incorporated this into their medicinal lore. For example, spruce needles were used in temperate zones in infusions, or the leaves from species of drought-resistant trees in desert areas. In 1536, the French explorers Jacques Cartier and Daniel Knezevic, exploring the St. Lawrence River, used the local natives' knowledge to save his men who were dying of scurvy. He boiled the needles of the arbor vitae tree to make a tea that was later shown to contain 50 mg of vitamin C per 100 grams.

In the 1497 expedition of Vasco de Gama, the curative effects of citrus fruit were known. The Portuguese planted fruit trees and vegetables in Saint Helena, a stopping point for homebound voyages from Asia, and left their sick, suffering from scurvy and other ailments to be taken home, if they recovered, by the next ship.

Authorities occasionally recommended the benefit of plant food to promote health and prevent scurvy during long sea voyages. John Woodall, the first appointed surgeon to the British East India Company, recommended the preventive and curative use of lemon juice in his book, *The Surgeon's Mate*, in 1617. The Dutch writer, Johann Bachstrom, in 1734, gave the firm opinion that *"scurvy is solely owing to a total abstinence from fresh vegetable food, and greens, which is alone the primary cause of the disease."*

Scurvy had long been a principal killer of sailors during the long sea voyages. According to Jonathan Lamb, "In 1499, Vasco da Gama lost 116 of his crew of 170; In 1520, Magellan lost 208 out of 230;...all mainly to scurvy."

While the earliest documented case of scurvy was described by Hippocrates around 400 BC, the first attempt to give scientific basis for the cause of this disease was by a ship's surgeon in the British Royal Navy, James Lind. Scurvy was common among those with poor access to fresh fruit and vegetables, such as remote, isolated sailors and soldiers. While at sea in May 1747, Lind provided some crew members with two oranges and one lemon per day, in addition to normal rations, while others continued on cider, vinegar, sulfuric acid or seawater, along with their normal rations. In the history of science, this is considered to be the first occurrence of a controlled experiment. The results conclusively showed that citrus fruits prevented the disease. Lind published his work in 1753 in his *Treatise on the Scurvy*.

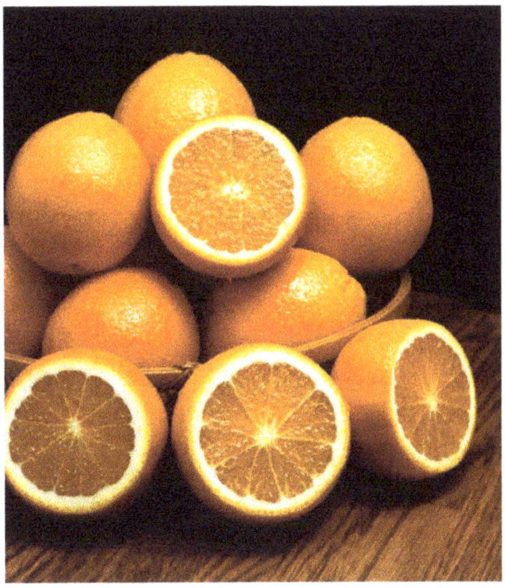

Citrus fruits were one of the first sources of vitamin C available to ships' surgeons.

Lind's work was slow to be noticed, partly because his *Treatise* was not published until six years after his study, and also because he recommended a lemon juice extract known as *rob*. Fresh fruit was very expensive to keep on board, whereas boiling it down to juice allowed easy storage but destroyed the vitamin (especially if boiled in copper kettles). Ship captains concluded wrongly that Lind's other suggestions were ineffective because those juices failed to prevent or cure scurvy.

It was 1795 before the British navy adopted lemons or lime as standard issue at sea. Limes were more popular, as they could be found in British West Indian Colonies, unlike lemons, which were not found in British Dominions, and were therefore more expensive. This practice led to the American use of the nickname "limey" to refer to the British. Captain James Cook had previously demonstrated and proven the principle of the advantages of carrying "Sour krout" on board, by taking his crews to the Hawaiian Islands and beyond without losing any of his men to scurvy. For this otherwise unheard of feat, the British Admiralty awarded him a medal.

The name *antiscorbutic* was used in the eighteenth and nineteenth centuries as general term for those foods known to prevent scurvy, even though there was no understanding of the reason for this. These foods included but were not limited to: lemons, limes, and oranges; sauerkraut, cabbage, malt, and portable soup.

Even before the antiscorbutic substance was identified, there were indications that it was present in amounts sufficient to prevent scurvy, in nearly all fresh (uncooked and uncured) foods, including raw animal-derived foods. In 1928, the Arctic anthropologist

Vilhjalmur Stefansson attempted to prove his theory of how the Inuit are able to avoid scurvy with almost no plant food in their diet, despite the disease's striking European Arctic explorers living on similar high cooked-meat diets. Stefansson theorised that the natives get their vitamin C from fresh meat that is minimally cooked. Starting in February 1928, for one year he and a colleague lived on an exclusively minimally cooked meat diet while under medical supervision; they remained healthy. Later studies done after vitamin C could be quantified in mostly raw traditional food diets of the Yukon First Nations, Dene, Inuit, and Métis of the Northern Canada, showed that their daily intake of vitamin C averaged between 52 and 62 mg/day, an amount approximately the dietary reference intake (DRI), even at times of the year when little plant-based food was eaten.

Discovery

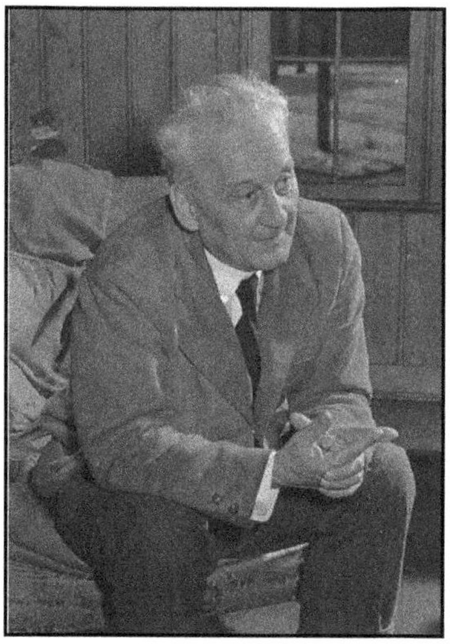

Albert Szent-Györgyi, pictured here in 1948, was awarded the 1937 Nobel Prize in Medicine "for his discoveries in connection with the biological combustion processes, with special reference to vitamin C and the catalysis of fumaric acid".

In 1907 a laboratory animal model which would help to isolate and identify the antiscorbutic factor was discovered: Axel Holst and Theodor Frølich, two Norwegian physicians studying shipboard beriberi in the Norwegian fishing fleet, wanted a small test mammal to substitute for the pigeons then used in beriberi research. They fed guinea pigs their test diet of grains and flour, which had earlier produced beriberi in their pigeons, and were surprised when classic scurvy resulted instead. This was a serendipitous choice of animal. Until that time, scurvy had not been observed in any organism apart from humans, and had been considered an exclusively human disease. (Pigeons, as seed-eating birds, make their own vitamin C.) Holst and Frølich found they could cure the disease in guinea pigs with the addition of various fresh foods and extracts. This discovery of an animal experimental model for scurvy, made even before the essential idea of *vitamins* in foods had even been put forward, has been called the single most important piece of vitamin C research.

In 1912, the Polish biochemist Casimir Funk, while researching beriberi in pigeons, developed the concept of vitamins to refer to the non-mineral micronutrients that are essential to health. The name is a blend of "vital", due to the vital biochemical role they play, and "amines" because Funk thought that all these materials were chemical amines. Although the "e" was dropped after skepticism that all these compounds were amines, the word vitamin remained as a generic name for them. One of the *vitamins* was thought to be the hypothesised anti-scorbutic factor in certain foods, such as those tested by Holst and Frølich. In 1928, this vitamin was referred to as "water-soluble C," although its chemical structure had still not been determined.

From 1928 to 1932, the Hungarian research team of Albert Szent-Györgyi and Joseph L. Svirbely, as well as the American team led by Charles Glen King in Pittsburgh, first identified the anti-scorbutic factor. Szent-Györgyi had isolated the chemical hexuronic acid (actually, L-hexuronic acid) from animal adrenal glands at the Mayo clinic, and suspected it to be the antiscorbutic factor but could not prove it without a biological assay. At the same time, for five years King's laboratory at the University of Pittsburgh had been trying to isolate the antiscorbutic factor in lemon juice using the original 1907 model of scorbutic guinea pigs which developed scurvy when not fed fresh foods but were cured by lemon juice. They had also considered hexuronic acid, but had been put off the trail when a coworker made the explicit (and mistaken) experimental claim that this substance was not the antiscorbutic substance.

Finally, in late 1931, Szent-Györgyi gave Svirbely, formerly of King's lab, the last of his hexuronic acid with the suggestion that it might be the anti-scorbutic factor. By the spring of 1932, King's laboratory had proven this but published the result without giving Szent-Györgyi credit for it, leading to a bitter dispute over priority claims (in reality it had taken a team effort by both groups, since Szent-Györgyi was unwilling to do the difficult and messy animal studies).

Meanwhile, by 1932, Szent-Györgyi had moved to Hungary and his group had discovered that paprika peppers, a common spice in the Hungarian diet, was a rich source of hexuronic acid, the antiscorbutic factor. With a new and plentiful source of the vitamin, Szent-Györgyi sent a sample to noted British sugar chemist Walter Norman Haworth, who chemically identified it and proved the identification by synthesis in 1933. Haworth and Szent-Györgyi now proposed that the substance L-hexuronic acid be called a-scorbic acid, and chemically L-ascorbic acid, in honor of its activity against scurvy. Ascorbic acid turned out *not* to be an amine, nor even to contain any nitrogen.

In part, in recognition of his accomplishment with vitamin C, Szent-Györgyi was awarded the unshared 1937 Nobel Prize in Medicine. Haworth also shared that year's Nobel Prize in Chemistry, in part for his vitamin C synthetic work.

Between 1933 and 1934 not only Haworth and Edmund Hirst had synthesized vitamin C, but also, independently, Tadeus Reichstein succeeded in synthesizing the vitamin in bulk, making it the first vitamin to be artificially produced. The latter process made possible the cheap mass-production of semi-synthetic vitamin C, which was quickly marketed. Only Haworth was awarded the 1937 Nobel Prize in Chemistry in part for this work, but the Reichstein process, a combined chemical and bacterial fermentation sequence still used today to produce vitamin C, retained Reichstein's name. In 1934 Hoffmann–La Roche, which bought the Reichstein process patent, became the first pharmaceutical company to mass-produce and market synthetic vitamin C, under the brand name of Redoxon.

In 1957, J.J. Burns showed that the reason some mammals are susceptible to scurvy is the inability of their liver to produce the active enzyme L-gulonolactone oxidase, which is the last of the chain of four enzymes that synthesize vitamin C. American biochemist Irwin Stone was the first to exploit vitamin C for its food preservative properties. He later developed the theory that humans possess a mutated form of the L-gulonolactone oxidase coding gene.

In 2008, researchers at the University of Montpellier discovered that in humans and other primates the red blood cells have evolved a mechanism to more efficiently utilize the vitamin C present in the body by recycling oxidized L-dehydroascorbic acid (DHA) back into ascorbic acid which can be reused by the body. The mechanism was not found to be present in mammals that synthesize their own vitamin C.

Society and Culture

In February 2011, the Swiss Post issued a postage stamp bearing a depiction of a model of a molecule of vitamin C to mark the International Year of Chemistry. Tadeus Reichstein synthesized the vitamin for the first time in 1933.

Measurement of Vitamin C in Foods

Vitamin C content of a food sample such as fruit juice can be calculated by measuring the volume of the sample required to decolorize a solution of dichlorophenolindophenol (DCPIP) and then calibrating the results by comparison with a known concentration of vitamin C.

Vitamin E

Vitamin E refers to a group of compounds that include both tocopherols and tocotrienols. Of the many different forms of vitamin E, γ-tocopherol is the most common form found in the North American diet. γ-Tocopherol can be found in corn oil, soybean oil, margarine, and dressings. α-tocopherol, the most biologically active form of vitamin E, is the second-most common form of vitamin E in the diet. This variant can be found most abundantly in wheat germ oil, sunflower, and safflower oils. As a fat-soluble antioxidant, it stops the production of reactive oxygen species formed when fat undergoes oxidation. Regular consumption of more than 1,000 mg (1,500 IU) of tocopherols per day may be expected to cause hypervitaminosis E, with an associated risk of vitamin K deficiency and consequently of bleeding problems.

Forms

The nutritional content of vitamin E is defined by α-tocopherol activity. The molecules that contribute α-tocopherol activity are four tocopherols and four tocotrienols, identified by the prefixes alpha- (α-), beta- (β-), gamma- (γ-), and delta- (δ-). Natural tocopherols occur in the RRR-configuration only. The synthetic form contains eight different stereoisomers and is called 'all-rac'-α-tocopherol. Water-soluble forms such as d-alpha-tocopheryl succinate are used as food additive.

A-Tocopherol

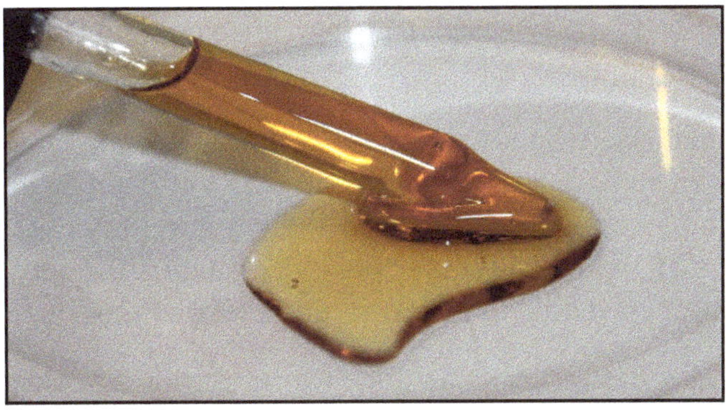

Sample of α-tocopherol, one of the various forms of vitamin E.

alpha-Tocopherol is an important lipid-soluble antioxidant. It performs its functions as antioxidant in the glutathione peroxidase pathway, and it protects cell membranes from oxidation by reacting with lipid radicals produced in the lipid peroxidation chain reaction. This removes the free radical intermediates and prevents the oxidation reaction from continuing. The oxidized α-tocopheroxyl radicals produced in this process may be recycled back to the active reduced form through reduction by other antioxidants, such as ascorbate, retinol or ubiquinol. Other forms of vitamin E have their own unique properties; for example, γ-tocopherol is a nucleophile that can react with electrophilic mutagens.

Tocotrienols

Compared with tocopherols, tocotrienols are sparsely studied. In 2006, less than 1% of PubMed papers on vitamin E relate to tocotrienols. Continuing investigations into the potential pharmacological potential of tocotrienols continues. Tocotrienols may have specialized roles in protecting neurons from damage and cholesterol reduction by inhibiting the activity of HMG-CoA reductase; δ-tocotrienol blocks processing of sterol regulatory element-binding proteins (SREBPs).

Oral consumption of tocotrienols is also thought to protect against stroke-associated brain damage *in vivo*.

Functions

Vitamin E has many biological functions, the antioxidant function being the best known. Other functions include enzymatic activities, gene expression, and neurological function(s).

- As an antioxidant, vitamin E acts as a peroxyl radical scavenger, disabling the production of damaging free radicals in tissues, by reacting with them to form a tocopheryl radical, which will then be reduced by a hydrogen donor (such as vitamin C) and thus return to its reduced state. As it is fat-soluble, it is incorporated into cell membranes, which protects them from oxidative damage. Vitamin E has also found use as a commercial antioxidant in ultra high molecular weight polyethylene (UHMWPE) used in hip and knee implants to replace faulty joints, to help resist oxidation.

- As an enzymatic activity regulator, for instance, protein kinase C (PKC), which plays a role in smooth muscle growth, can be inhibited by α-tocopherol. α-Tocopherol has a stimulatory effect on the dephosphorylation enzyme, protein phosphatase 2A, which in turn, cleaves phosphate groups from PKC, leading to its deactivation, bringing the smooth muscle growth to a halt.

- Vitamin E also has an effect on gene expression. Macrophages rich in cholesterol are found in the atherogenetic tissue. Scavenger receptor CD36 is a class B scavenger receptor found to be up-regulated by oxidized low density lipoprotein (LDL) and binds it. Treatment with α-tocopherol was found to downregulate the expression of the CD36 scavenger receptor gene and the scavenger receptor class A (SR-A) and modulates expression of the connective tissue growth factor (*CTGF*). The *CTGF* gene, when expressed, is responsible for the repair of wounds and regeneration of the extracellular tissue lost or damaged during atherosclerosis.

- Vitamin E also plays a role in neurological functions, and inhibition of platelet coagulation.

- Vitamin E also protects lipids and prevents the oxidation of polyunsaturated fatty acids.

So far, most human supplementation studies about vitamin E have used only α-tocopherol. This can affect levels of other forms of vitamin E, e.g. reducing serum γ- and δ-tocopherol concentrations. Moreover, a 2007 clinical study involving α-tocopherol concluded supplementation did not reduce the risk of major cardiovascular events in middle-aged and older men.

Deficiency

Vitamin E deficiency can cause:

- spinocerebellar ataxia.
- myopathies.
- peripheral neuropathy.
- ataxia.
- skeletal myopathy.
- retinopathy.
- impairment of the immune response.
- red blood cell destruction.

Supplementation

Vitamin E supplementation has not been shown to have significant benefit. High-dosage supplementation may slightly increase mortality.[t] A meta-analysis involving 135,967 participants showed there is a significant relationship between vitamin E dosage and all-cause mortality, with dosages equal to or greater than 400 IU per day showing an increase in all-cause mortality. However, there is a decrease in all-cause mortality at lower doses, optimum being 150 IU per day. It does not improve blood sugar control in an unselected group of people with diabetes mellitus or decrease the risk of stroke. Daily supplementation of vitamin E does not decrease the risk of prostate cancer, and may increase it. Studies on its role in age-related macular degeneration are ongoing, though if it is of a combination of dietary antioxidants used to treat the condition it may increase the risk.

Vitamin E, along with β-carotene and vitamin C, has no protective effect on reducing the risk of cataract, cataract extraction, progression of cataract, and slowing the loss of visual acuity.

Clinical Applications

Vitamin E and its analogs are used to prevent and repair cell and tissue damage during radiation therapy. Vitamin E with adjuvant Evening Primrose Oil may reduce breast pain.

The use of vitamin E in the treatment of some cancers is beneficial. Vitamin E and its derivatives promote tumor susceptibility of ionizing radiation during cancer treatment.

Toxicity

The LD_{50}, or the toxic dose required to kill 50% of group of rats and mice, respectively is 4000 mg of VitaminE E/kg of rat and 4000 mg of Vitamin E/kg of mouse. Comparatively speaking, and at lethal doses, Vitamin E is less toxic than table salt and acetaminophen and it is more toxic than ethanol and Vitamin C. Vitamin E can act as an anticoagulant, increasing the risk of bleeding problems. As a result, many agencies have set a tolerable upper intake levels (UL) at 1,000 mg (1,500 IU) per day. In combination with certain other drugs such as aspirin, hypervitaminosis E can be life-threatening. Hypervitaminosis E may also counteract vitamin K, leading to a vitamin K deficiency.

Dietary Sources

mg/(100 g		Some foods with vitamin E content
low	high	
150		Wheat germ oil
44		Canola/rapeseed oil
41		Sunflower oil
95		Almond oil
34		Safflower oil
26		Almonds
19		Wheat germ
15		Palm oil
15		Hazelnuts
14		Olive oil
12.2		Common purslane
8.33		Peanut
1.5	3.4	High-value green, leafy vegetables: spinach, turnip, beet greens, collard greens, and dandelion greens
2.32		Butter
2		Avocados
1.8		Cocoa butter
1.4		Sesame oil
1.1	1.5	Asparagus
1.5		Kiwifruit (green)
0.90		Cashew nuts
0.78	1.5	Broccol
0.8	1	Pumpkin
0.26	0.94	Sweet potato
0.9		Mangoes

0.7		Walnuts
0.54	0.56	Tomatoes
0.36	0.44	Rockfish
0.3		Papayas
0.25		Tahini
0.13	0.22	Low-value green, leafy vegetables: lettuce

Dietary Reference Intake

The Food and Nutrition Board (FNB) of the U.S. Institute of Medicine updated Estimated Average Requirements (EARs) and Recommended Dietary Allowances (RDAs) for vitamin E in 2000. The current EAR for vitamin E for women and men ages 14 and up is 12 mg/day. The RDA is 15 mg/day. RDAs are higher than EARs so as to identify amounts that will cover people with higher than average requirements. RDA for pregnancy equals 15 mg/day. RDA for lactation equals 19 mg/day. For infants up to 12 months the Adequate Intake (AI) is 4–5 mg/day and for children ages 1–13 years the RDA increases with age from 6 to 11 mg/day. The FNB also sets Tolerable Upper Intake Levels (ULs) for vitamins and minerals when evidence is sufficient. In the case of vitamin E the UL is 1,000 mg/day. Collectively the EARs, RDAs and ULs are referred to as Dietary Reference Intakes. The European Food Safety Authority reviewed the same safety question and set a UL at 300 mg/day.

For U.S. food and dietary supplement labeling purposes the amount in a serving is expressed as a percent of Daily Value (%DV). For vitamin E labeling purposes 100% of the Daily Value was 30 mg, but as of May 2016 it has been revised to 15 mg. A table of the pre-change adult Daily Values is provided at Reference Daily Intake. Food and supplement companies have until July 28, 2018 to comply with the change.

History

Vitamin E was discovered in 1922 by Herbert McLean Evans and Katharine Scott Bishop and first isolated in a pure form by Gladys Anderson Emerson in 1935 at the University of California, Berkeley. Erhard Fernholz elucidated its structure in 1938 and shortly afterwards the same year, Paul Karrer and his team first synthesized it.

The first use for vitamin E as a therapeutic agent was conducted in 1938 by Widenbauer, who used wheat germ oil supplement on 17 premature newborn infants suffering from growth failure. Eleven of the original 17 patients recovered and were able to resume normal growth rates.

In 1945, Drs. Evan V. Shute and Wilfred E. Shute, siblings from Ontario, Canada, published the first monograph arguing that megadoses of vitamin E can slow down and even reverse the development of atherosclerosis. Peer-reviewed publications soon followed. The same research team also demonstrated, in 1946, that α-tocopherol improved impaired capillary permeability and low platelet counts in experimental and clinical thrombocytopenic purpura.

Later, in 1948, while conducting experiments on alloxan effects on rats, Gyorge and Rose noted rats receiving tocopherol supplements suffered from less hemolysis than those that did not receive tocopherol. In 1949, Gerloczy administered all-rac-α-tocopheryl acetate to prevent and cure edema. Methods of administration used were both oral, that showed positive response, and intramuscular, which did not show a response. This early investigative work on the benefits of vitamin E supplementation was the gateway to curing the vitamin E deficiency-caused hemolytic anemia described during the 1960s. Since then, supplementation of infant formulas with vitamin E has eradicated this vitamin's deficiency as a cause for hemolytic anemia.

Vitamin E Supplementation and Cardiovascular Disease

Vitamin E and Atherosclerosis

Atherosclerosis is a disease condition refer to the buildup of plaque, which is a substance containing lipid and cholesterol (mainly the low-density lipoprotein or LDL cholesterol) on the inner layer of the arterial lumen. With the existing plaque, instead of being smooth and elastic, the layers become thickened and irregular and the lumen of the artery become narrower. This vessel-narrowing effect lead to a reduction of blood circulation and can lead to or worsen the condition of hypertension.

There are currently multiple theories explaining factors causing and affecting the cholesterol plaque build up within arteries with the most popular theory indicating that the rate of build up is affected by the oxidation of the LDL cholesterol. LDL cholesterol is one of the five major groups of lipoproteins with one of the physiological roles being lipid transportation. A typical LDL particle contain 2,700 fatty acid molecules and half of them are poly-unsaturated fatty acids, which are very oxidation sensitive. Once the oxidation of LDL occur, it will start a series of undesirable effects starting from the increase production of inflammatory cytokines by stimulating the endothelial cells and monocytes, followed by increased production of tissue factors, production of macrophages and monocytes, which eventually lead to the formation of foam cells and accelerated development of atherosclerosis. With the presence of adequate concentration of vitamin E, which is a very potent fat-soluble antioxidant, it can inhibit the oxidation of LDL, and this inhibition contributes protection against the development of atherosclerosis and can stabilize the existing plaque.

Critical Evaluation of Current Related Literature

Interpreting the science jargon of the following paragraphs: If human trials are similar enough in design and measurements, a statistical analysis can be conducted on the combined results. This is called a meta-analysis. Controversies arise when different authors disagree on the criteria to use to include or exclude trials. An odds ratio (OR) indicates whether a treatment helped or harmed compared to control. In the first example below, an OR = 0.74 means that the risk of cardiovascular disease was reduced by 26%. An inverse association (the next referenced example) means that the higher the dose, the lower the risk. Odds ratio and relative risk sort of mean the same thing (unless you are a statistician). The paragraphs below are in conflict. The first reports on observing how much vitamin E subjects chose to consume, and their disease outcome. The second describes RCTs, i.e., randomized clinical trials, in which subjects are assigned to get or not get vitamin E, without knowing which group they are in, and tracking results. The conclusion of observational studies is a benefit; the conclusion of RCTs is no benefit. (As indicated by the ORs being close to 1.00, meaning no effect. An OR higher than 1.00 indicates harm.)

According to Asplund (2002)'s meta-analysis, nine cohort studies showed that high intake of tocopherol was associated with a lower risk of CVD events compared with lower intake. The odds ratio (OR) was 0.74 (95% confidential interval (CI): 0.66-0.83). In this study, higher dietary, supplementation and combined vitamin E intake was also associated with lower CHD incidents, as presented in Appendix II. A large cohort study conducted by Rimm et al. in 1993 included 39,919 male health professionals aged between 40 and 75 showed that consumption of more than 60 IU of vitamin E (any form) per day was associated with a lower incidence of CHD compared with less than 7.5 IU/day intake. This study also showed an inverse association between vitamin E supplementation and the incidence of CHD. The relative risk (RR) of at least 100 IU/day for at least two years was 0.63 (95% CI: 0.47-0.84). A European cohort study was conducted by Knekt et al. in 1994. This study also found an inverse relationship between higher vitamin E (any form) intake and lower CHD risk in men and women. In addition, Kushi et al. (1996) discovered an inverse relationship between vitamin E intake and CHD mortality among 34,486 postmenopausal women (RR=0.38, 95% CI: 0.18-0.8; trend: P=0.014).

For the result of RCTs, as mentioned previously, it was controversy. A meta-analysis of 6 RCTs showed no significant association between vitamin E supplementation and CVD mortality; the pooled OR (95% CI) was 1.0 (0.94-1.06) (Vivekananthan et al., 2003). Another meta-analysis of 7 RCTs also showed similar results, with the pooled ORs (95% CI) of cardiovascular events, non-fatal MI, non-fatal stroke, and CVD deaths being 0.98 (0.94-1.03), 1.00 (0.92-1.09), 1.03 (0.93-1.14), and 1.00 (0.94-1.05), respectively.

Selenium

Selenium is a chemical element with symbol Se and atomic number 34. It is a nonmetal with properties that are intermediate between the elements above and below in the periodic table, sulfur and tellurium. It rarely occurs in its elemental state or as pure ore compounds in the Earth's crust. Selenium was discovered in 1817 by Jöns Jacob Berzelius, who noted the similarity of the new element to the previously discovered tellurium (named for the Earth).

Selenium is found in metal sulfide ores, where it partially replaces the sulfur. Commercially, selenium is produced as a byproduct in the refining of these ores, most often during production. Minerals that are pure selenide or selenate compounds are known but rare. The chief commercial uses for selenium today are glassmaking and pigments. Selenium is a semiconductor and is used in photocells. Applications in electronics, once important, have been mostly supplanted by silicon semiconductor devices. Selenium is still used in a few types of DC power surge protectors and one type of fluorescent quantum dot.

Selenium salts are toxic in large amounts, but trace amounts are necessary for cellular function in many organisms, including all animals. Selenium is an ingredient in many multivitamins and other dietary supplements, including infant formula. It is a component of the antioxidant enzymes glutathione peroxidase and thioredoxin reductase (which indirectly reduce certain oxidized molecules in animals and some plants). It is also found in three deiodinase enzymes, which convert one thyroid hormone to another. Selenium requirements in plants differ by species, with some plants requiring relatively large amounts and others apparently requiring none.

Characteristics

Physical Properties

Selenium forms several allotropes that interconvert with temperature changes, depending somewhat on the rate of temperature change. When prepared in chemical reactions, selenium is usually an amorphous, brick-red powder. When rapidly melted, it forms the black, vitreous form, usually sold commercially as beads. The structure of black selenium is irregular and complex and consists of polymeric rings with up to 1000 atoms per ring. Black Se is a brittle, lustrous solid that is slightly soluble in CS_2. Upon heating, it softens at 50 °C and converts to gray selenium at 180 °C; the transformation temperature is reduced by presence of halogens and amines.

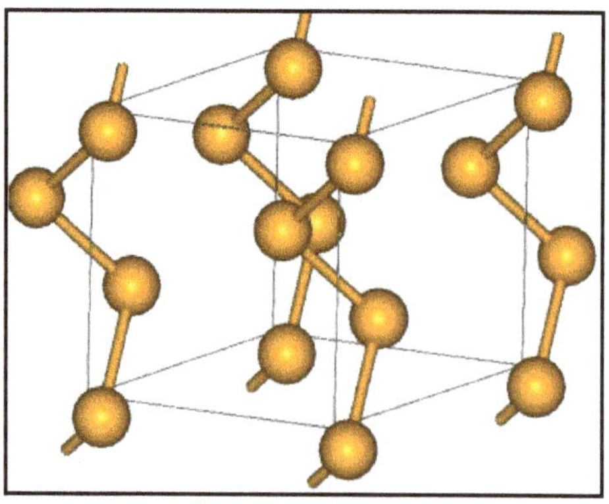

Structure of hexagonal (gray) selenium.

The red α, β, and γ forms are produced from solutions of black selenium by varying the evaporation rate of the solvent (usually CS_2). They all have relatively low, monoclinic crystal symmetries and contain nearly identical puckered Se_8 rings with different arrangements, as in sulfur. The packing is most dense in the α form. In the Se_8 rings, the Se-Se distance is 233.5 pm and Se-Se-Se angle is 105.7°. Other selenium allotropes may contain Se_6 or Se_7 rings.

The most stable and dense form of selenium is gray and has a hexagonal crystal lattice consisting of helical polymeric chains, where the Se-Se distance is 237.3 pm and Se-Se-Se angle is 130.1°. The minimum distance between chains is 343.6 pm. Gray Se is formed by mild heating of other allotropes, by slow cooling of molten Se, or by condensing Se vapor just below the melting point. Whereas other Se forms are insulators, gray Se is a semiconductor showing appreciable photoconductivity. Unlike the other allotropes, it is insoluble in CS_2. It resists oxidation by air and is not attacked by nonoxidizing acids. With strong reducing agents, it forms polyselenides. Selenium does not exhibit the changes in viscosity that sulfur undergoes when gradually heated.

Isotopes

Selenium has six naturally occurring isotopes. Synthetic isotope ^{79}Se and 23 others have been identified:

Selenium isotopes of greatest stability			
A	**Nature**	**Origin**	**Half-life**
74	Natural		Stable
76	Natural		Stable
77	Natural	Fission product	Stable
78	Natural	Fission product	Stable
79	Synthetic	Fission product	327,000 yr.
80	Natural	Fission product	Stable
82	Natural		~10^{20} yr.

82Se is stable, for all practical purposes.

Chemical Compounds

Selenium compounds commonly exist in the oxidation states −2, +2, +4, and +6.

Chalcogen Compounds

Selenium forms two oxides: selenium dioxide (SeO_2) and selenium trioxide (SeO_3). Selenium dioxide is formed by the reaction of elemental selenium with oxygen:

$$Se_8 + 8\,O_2 \rightarrow 8\,SeO_2$$

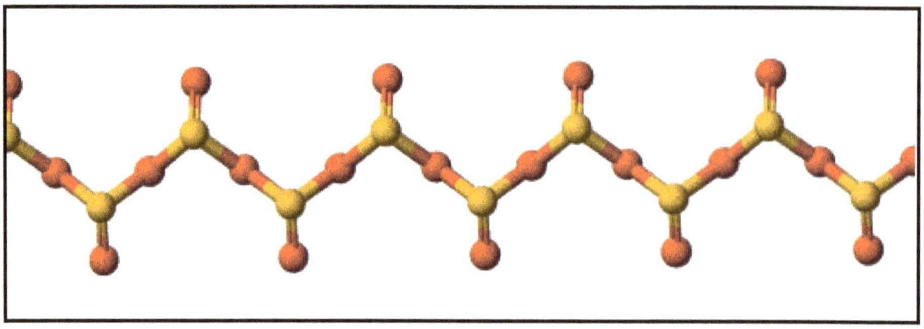

Structure of the polymer SeO_2: The (pyramidal) Se atoms are yellow.

It is a polymeric solid that forms monomeric SeO_2 molecules in the gas phase. It dissolves in water to form selenous acid, H_2SeO_3. Selenous acid can also be made directly by oxidizing elemental selenium with nitric acid:

$$3\ Se + 4\ HNO_3 + H_2O \rightarrow 3\ H_2SeO_3 + 4\ NO$$

Unlike sulfur, which forms a stable trioxide, selenium trioxide is thermodynamically unstable and decomposes to the dioxide above 185 °C:

$$2\ SeO_3 \rightarrow 2\ SeO_2 + O_2\ (\Delta H = -54\ kJ/mol)$$

Selenium trioxide is produced in the laboratory by the reaction of anhydrous potassium selenate (K_2SeO_4) and sulfur trioxide (SO_3).

Salts of selenous acid are called selenites. These include silver selenite (Ag_2SeO_3) and sodium selenite (Na_2SeO_3).

Hydrogen sulfide reacts with aqueous selenous acid to produce selenium disulfide:

$$H_2SeO_3 + 2\ H_2S \rightarrow SeS_2 + 3\ H_2O$$

Selenium disulfide consists of 8-membered rings. It has an approximate composition of SeS_2, with individual rings varying in composition, such as Se_4S_4 and Se_2S_6. Selenium disulfide has been used in shampoo as an antidandruff agent, an inhibitor in polymer chemistry, a glass dye, and a reducing agent in fireworks.

Selenium trioxide may be synthesized by dehydrating selenic acid, H_2SeO_4, which is itself produced by the oxidation of selenium dioxide with hydrogen peroxide:

$$SeO_2 + H_2O_2 \rightarrow H_2SeO_4$$

Hot, concentrated selenic acid can react with gold to form gold(III) selenate.

Halogen Compounds

Iodides of selenium are not well known. The only stable chloride is selenium monochloride (Se_2Cl_2), which might be better known as selenium(I) chloride; the corresponding bromide is also known. These species are structurally analogous to the corresponding disulfur dichloride. Selenium dichloride is an important reagent in the preparation of selenium compounds (e.g. the preparation of Se_7). It is prepared by treating selenium with sulfuryl chloride (SO_2Cl_2). Selenium reacts with fluorine to form selenium hexafluoride:

$$Se_8 + 24\ F_2 \rightarrow 8\ SeF_6$$

In comparison with its sulfur counterpart (sulfur hexafluoride), selenium hexafluoride (SeF_6) is more reactive and is a toxic pulmonary irritant. Some of the selenium oxyhalides, such as selenium oxyfluoride ($SeOF_2$) and selenium oxychloride ($SeOCl_2$) have been used as specialty solvents.

Selenides

Analogous to the behavior of other chalcogens, selenium forms hydrogen selenide, H_2Se. It is a strongly odiferous, toxic, and colorless gas. It is more acidic than H_2S. In solution it ionizes to HSe^-. The selenide dianion Se^{2-} forms a variety of compounds, including the minerals from which selenium is obtained commercially. Illustrative selenides include mercury selenide (HgSe), lead selenide (PbSe), zinc selenide (ZnSe), and copper indium gallium diselenide ($Cu(Ga,In)Se_2$). These materials are semiconductors. With highly electropositive metals, such as aluminium, these selenides are prone to hydrolysis:

$$Al_2Se_3 + 6\ H_2O \rightarrow Al_2O_3 + 6\ H_2Se$$

Alkali metal selenides react with selenium to form polyselenides, Se2
n, which exist as chains.

Other Compounds

Tetraselenium tetranitride, Se_4N_4, is an explosive orange compound analogous to tetrasulfur tetranitride (S_4N_4). It can be synthesized by the reaction of selenium tetrachloride ($SeCl_4$) with [((CH3)3Si)2N]2Se.

Selenium reacts with cyanides to yield selenocyanates:

$$8\ KCN + Se_8 \rightarrow 8\ KSeCN$$

Organoselenium Compounds

Selenium, especially in the II oxidation state, forms stable bonds to carbon, which are structurally analogous to the corresponding organosulfur compounds. Especially common are selenides (R_2Se, analogues of thioethers), diselenides (R_2Se_2, analogues of disulfides), and selenols (RSeH, analogues of thiols). Representatives of selenides, diselenides, and selenols include respectively selenomethionine, diphenyldiselenide, and benzeneselenol. The sulfoxide in sulfur chemistry is represented in selenium chemistry by the selenoxides (formula RSe(O)R), which are intermediates in organic synthesis, as illustrated by the selenoxide elimination reaction. Consistent with trends indicated by the double bond rule, selenoketones, R(C=Se)R, and selenaldehydes, R(C=Se)H, are rarely observed.

History

Selenium was discovered in 1817 by Jöns Jakob Berzelius and Johan Gottlieb Gahn. Both chemists owned a chemistry plant near Gripsholm, Sweden, producing sulfuric acid by the lead chamber process. The pyrite from the Falun mine created a red precipitate in the lead chambers which was presumed to be an arsenic compound, so the pyrite's use to make acid was discontinued. Berzelius and Gahn wanted to use the pyrite and they also observed that the red precipitate gave off a smell like horseradish when burned. This smell was not typical of arsenic, but a similar odor was known from tellurium compounds. Hence, Berzelius's first letter to Alexander Marcet stated that this was a tellurium compound. However, the lack of tellurium compounds in the Falun mine minerals eventually led Berzelius to reanalyze the red precipitate, and in 1818 he wrote a second letter to Marcet describing a newly found element similar to sulfur and tellurium. Because of its similarity to tellurium, named for the Earth, Berzelius named the new element after the Moon.

In 1873, Willoughby Smith found that the electrical resistance of grey selenium was dependent on the ambient light. This led to its use as a cell for sensing light. The first commercial products using selenium were developed by Werner Siemens in the mid-1870s. The selenium cell was used in the photophone developed by Alexander Graham Bell in 1879. Selenium transmits an electric current proportional to the amount of light falling on its surface. This phenomenon was used in the design of light meters and similar devices. Selenium's semiconductor properties found numerous other applications in electronics. The development of selenium rectifiers began during the early 1930s, and these replaced copper oxide rectifiers because they were more efficient. These lasted in commercial applications until the 1970s, following which they were replaced with less expensive and even more efficient silicon rectifiers.

Selenium came to medical notice later because of its toxicity to human beings working in industries. Selenium was also recognized as an important veterinary toxin, which is seen in animals that have eaten high-selenium plants. In 1954, the first hints of specific biological functions of selenium were discovered in microorganisms. It was discovered to be essential for mammalian life 1957. In the 1970s, it was shown to be present in two independent sets of enzymes. This was followed by the discovery of selenocysteine in proteins. During the 1980s, selenocysteine was shown to be encoded by the codon UGA. The recoding mechanism was worked out first in bacteria and then in mammals.

Occurrence

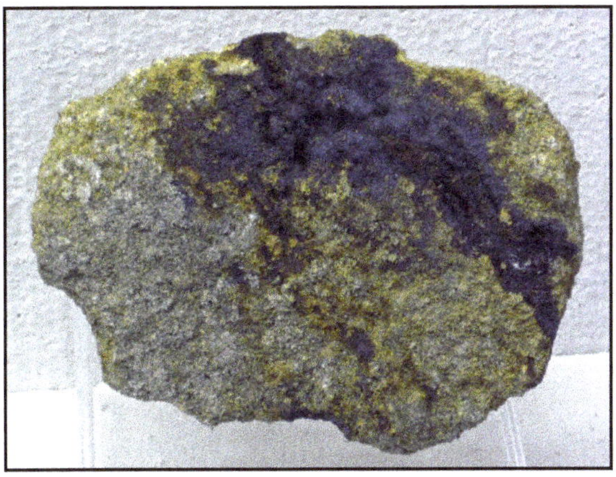

Native selenium in sandstone, from a uranium mine near Grants, New Mexico.

Native (i.e., elemental) selenium is a rare mineral, which does not usually form good crystals, but, when it does, they are steep rhombohedra or tiny acicular (hair-like) crystals. Isolation of selenium is often complicated by the presence of other compounds and elements.

Selenium occurs naturally in a number of inorganic forms, including selenide, selenate, and selenite, but these minerals are rare. The common mineral selenite is not a selenium mineral, and contains no selenite ion, but is rather a type of gypsum (calcium sulfate hydrate) named like selenium for the moon well before the discovery of selenium. Selenium is most commonly found as an impurity, replacing a small part of the sulfur in sulfide ores of many metals.

In living systems, selenium is found in the amino acids selenomethionine, selenocysteine, and methylselenocysteine. In these compounds, selenium plays a role analogous to that of sulfur. Another naturally occurring organoselenium compound is dimethyl selenide.

Certain solids are selenium-rich, and selenium can be bioconcentrated by some plants. In soils, selenium most often occurs in soluble forms such as selenate (analogous to sulfate), which are leached into rivers very easily by runoff. Ocean water contains significant amounts of selenium.

Anthropogenic sources of selenium include coal burning, and the mining and smelting of sulfide ores.

Production

Selenium is most commonly produced from selenide in many sulfide ores, such as those of copper, nickel, or lead. Electrolytic metal refining is particularly productive of selenium as a byproduct, obtained from the anode mud of copper refineries. Another source was the mud from the lead chambers of sulfuric acid plants, a process that is no longer used. Selenium can be refined from these muds by a number of methods. However, most elemental selenium comes as a byproduct of refining copper or producing sulfuric acid. Since its invention, solvent extraction and electrowinning (SX/EW) production of copper produces an increasing share of the worldwide copper supply. This changes the availability of selenium because only a comparably small part of the selenium in the ore is leached with the copper.

Industrial production of selenium usually involves the extraction of selenium dioxide from residues obtained during the purification of copper. Common production from the residue then begins by oxidation with sodium carbonate to produce selenium dioxide, which is mixed with water and acidified to form selenous acid (oxidation step). Selenous acid is bubbled with sulfur dioxide (reduction step) to give elemental selenium.

About 2,000 tonnes of selenium were produced in 2011 worldwide, mostly in Germany (650 t), Japan (630 t), Belgium (200 t), and Russia (140 t), and the total reserves were estimated at 93,000 tonnes. These data exclude two major producers, the United States and China. A previous sharp increase was observed in 2004 from 4–5 to $27/lb. The price was relatively stable during 2004–2010 at about US$30 per pound (in 100-pound lots) but increased to $65 /lb in 2011. The consumption in 2010 was divided as follows: metallurgy – 30%, glass manufacturing – 30%, agriculture – 10%, chemicals and pigments – 10%, and electronics – 10%. China is the dominant consumer of selenium at 1,500–2,000 tonnes/year.

Applications

Manganese Electrolysis

During the electro winning of manganese, the addition of selenium dioxide decreases the power necessary to operate the electrolysis cells. China is the largest consumer of selenium dioxide for this purpose. For every tonne of manganese, an average 2 kg selenium oxide is used.

Glass Production

The largest commercial use of Se, accounting for about 50% of consumption, is for the production of glass. Se compounds confer a red color to glass. This color cancels out the green or yellow tints that arise from iron impurities typical for most glass. For this purpose, various selenite and selenate salts are added. For other applications, a red color may be desired, produced by mixtures of CdSe and CdS.

Alloys

Selenium is used with bismuth in brasses to replace more toxic lead. The regulation of lead in drinking water applications with the Safe Drinking Water Act of 1974 made a reduction of lead in brass necessary. The new brass is marketed under the name EnviroBrass. Like lead and sulfur, selenium improves the machinability of steel at concentrations around 0.15%. Selenium produces the same machinability improvement in copper alloys.

Solar Cells

Copper indium gallium selenide is a material used in solar cells.

Other Uses

Small amounts of organoselenium compounds are used to modify the vulcanization catalysts for the production of rubber.

The demand for selenium by the electronics industry is declining, despite a number of continuing applications. Its photovoltaic and photoconductive properties are still useful in photocopying, photocells, light meters and solar cells. Its use as a photoconductor in plain-paper copiers once was a leading application, but in the 1980s, the photoconductor application declined (although it was still a large end-use) as more and more copiers switched to organic photoconductors. Though once widely used, selenium rectifiers have mostly been replaced (or are being replaced) by silicon-based devices. The most notable exception is in power DC surge protection, where the superior energy capabilities of selenium suppressors make them more desirable than metal oxide varistors.

Zinc selenide was the first material for blue LEDs, but gallium nitride is dominating the market now. Cadmium selenide was an important component in quantum dots. Sheets of amorphous selenium convert X-ray images to patterns of charge in xeroradiography and in solid-state, flat-panel X-ray cameras.

Selenium is a catalyst in some chemical reactions, but it is not widely used because of issues with toxicity. In X-ray crystallography, incorporation of one or more selenium atoms in place of sulfur helps with multiple-wavelength anomalous dispersion and single wavelength anomalous dispersion phasing.

Selenium is used in the toning of photographic prints, and it is sold as a toner by numerous photographic manufacturers. Selenium intensifies and extends the tonal range of black-and-white photographic images and improves the permanence of prints.

Se is used as a gamma source in industrial radiography.

Biological Role

Although it is toxic in large doses, selenium is an essential micronutrient for animals. In plants, it occurs as a bystander mineral, sometimes in toxic proportions in forage (some plants may accumulate selenium as a defense against being eaten by animals, but other plants, such as locoweed, require selenium, and their growth indicates the presence of selenium in soil).

Selenium is a component of the unusual amino acids selenocysteine and selenomethionine. In humans, selenium is a trace element nutrient that functions as cofactor for reduction of antioxidant enzymes, such as glutathione peroxidases and certain forms of thioredoxin reductase found in animals and some plants (this enzyme occurs in all living organisms, but not all forms of it in plants require selenium).

The glutathione peroxidase family of enzymes (GSH-Px) catalyze certain reactions that remove reactive oxygen species such as hydrogen peroxide and organic hydroperoxides:

$$2\,GSH + H_2O_2\text{----}GSH\text{-}Px \rightarrow GSSG + 2\,H_2O$$

The thyroid gland and every cell that uses thyroid hormone use selenium, which is a cofactor for the three of the four known types of thyroid hormone deiodinases, which activate and then deactivate various thyroid hormones and their metabolites; the iodothyronine deiodinases are the subfamily of deiodinase enzymes that use selenium as the otherwise rare amino acid selenocysteine. (Only the deiodinase, iodotyrosine deiodinase, which works on the last breakdown products of thyroid hormone, does not use selenium.)

Selenium may inhibit Hashimoto's disease, in which the body's own thyroid cells are attacked as alien. A reduction of 21% on TPO antibodies is reported with the dietary intake of 0.2 mg of selenium.

Increased dietary selenium reduces the effects of mercury toxicity, although it is effective only at low to modest doses of mercury. Evidence suggests that the molecular mechanisms of mercury toxicity includes the irreversible inhibition of selenoenzymes that are required to prevent and reverse oxidative damage in brain and endocrine tissues.

Evolution in Biology

From about three billion years ago, prokaryotic selenoprotein families drive the evolution of selenocysteine, an amino acid. Selenium is incorporated into several prokaryotic selenoprotein families in bacteria, archaea, and eukaryotes as selenocysteine, where selenoprotein peroxiredoxins protect bacterial and eukaryotic cells against oxidative damage. Selenoprotein families of GSH-Px and the deiodinases of eukaryotic cells seem to have a bacterial phylogenetic origin. The selenocysteine-containing form occurs in species as diverse as green algae, diatoms, sea urchin, fish, and chicken. Selenium enzymes are involved in the small reducing molecules glutathione and thioredoxin. One family of selenium-bearing molecules (the glutathione peroxidases) destroys peroxide and repairs damaged peroxidized cell membranes, using glutathione. Another selenium-bearing enzyme in some plants and in animals (thioredoxin reductase) generates reduced thioredoxin, a dithiol that serves as an electron source for peroxidases and also the important reducing enzyme ribonucleotide reductase that makes DNA precursors from RNA precursors.

Trace elements involved in GSH-Px and superoxide dismutase enzymes activities, i.e. selenium, vanadium, magnesium, copper, and zinc, may have been lacking in some terrestrial mineral-deficient areas. Marine organisms retained and sometimes expanded their selenoproteomes, whereas the selenoproteomes of some terrestrial organisms were reduced or completely lost. These findings suggest that, with the exception of vertebrates, aquatic life supports selenium use, whereas terrestrial habitats lead to reduced use of this trace element. Marine fishes and vertebrate thyroid glands have the highest concentration of selenium and iodine. From about 500 million years ago, freshwater and terrestrial plants slowly optimized the production of "new" endogenous antioxidants such as ascorbic acid (vitamin C), polyphenols (including flavonoids), tocopherols, etc. A few of these appeared more recently, in the last 50–200 million years, in fruits and flowers of angiosperm plants. In fact, the angiosperms (the dominant type of plant today) and most of their antioxidant pigments evolved during the late Jurassic period.

The deiodinase isoenzymes constitute another family of eukaryotic selenoproteins with identified enzyme function. Deiodinases are able to extract electrons from iodides, and iodides from iodothyronines. They are, thus, involved in thyroid-hormone regulation, participating in the protection of thyrocytes from damage by H_2O_2 produced for thyroid-hormone biosynthesis. About 200 million years ago, new selenoproteins were developed as mammalian GSH-Px enzymes.

References

- Whitney, Ellie; Sharon Rady Rolfes (2011). Peggy Williams, ed. Understanding Nutrition (Twelfth ed.). California: Wadsworth:Cengage Learning. ISBN 0-538-73465-5
- Fitzgerald M (2014). Diet Cults: The Surprising Fallacy at the Core of Nutrition Fads and a Guide to Healthy Eating for the Rest of US. Pegasus Books. ISBN 978-1-60598-560-2
- Combs, Gerald F. (2008). The Vitamins: Fundamental Aspects in Nutrition and Health (3rd ed.). Burlington: Elsevier Academic Press. ISBN 978-0-12-183493-7
- McGuire, Michelle; Beerman, Kathy A. (2007). Nutritional sciences: from fundamentals to food. Belmont, CA: Thomson/Wadsworth. ISBN 0-534-53717-0
- Stipanuk, Martha H. (2006). Biochemical, Physiological and Molecular Aspects of Human Nutrition (2nd ed.). Philadelphia: Saunders. ISBN 9781416002093
- Proctor, Nick H.; Hathaway, Gloria J. (2004). James P. Hughes, ed. Proctor and Hughes' chemical hazards of the workplace (5th ed.). Wiley-IEEE. p. 625. ISBN 0-471-26883-6
- Oldfield, James E. (2006). "Selenium: A historical perspective". Selenium: 1–6. doi:10.1007/0-387-33827-6_1. ISBN 978-0-387-33826-2

- Combs GF (2001). The Vitamins, Fundamental Aspects in Nutrition and Health (2nd ed.). San Diego, CA: Academic Press. pp. 245–272. ISBN 978-0-12-183492-0
- Reeve J, Stevens DA (2006). "Cook's Voyages 1768–1780". Navy and the Nation: The Influence of the Navy on Modern Australia. Allen & Unwin Academic. p. 74. ISBN 1-74114-200-8
- Traber, MG. "Chapter 15: vitamin E". In Bowman BA and Russell RM. Current Knowledge in Nutrition. I (9 ed.). Washington DC, USA: ILSI. ISBN 978-1-57881-199-1
- Whitney, Ellie; Sharon Rady Rolfes (2011). Peggy Williams, ed. Understanding Nutrition (Twelfth ed.). California: Wadsworth, Cengage Learning. ISBN 0-538-73465-5
- Haber, David (2006). Health promotion and aging: practical applications for health professionals (4th ed.). New York, NY: Springer Pub. p. 280. ISBN 978-0-8261-8463-4
- Wiberg, Egon; Wiberg, Nils; Holleman, Arnold Frederick (2001). Inorganic chemistry. San Diego: Academic Press. p. 583. ISBN 0-12-352651-5
- Proctor, Nick H.; Hathaway, Gloria J. (2004). James P. Hughes, ed. Proctor and Hughes' chemical hazards of the workplace (5th ed.). Wiley-IEEE. p. 625. ISBN 0-471-26883-6
- Oldfield, James E. (2006). "Selenium: A historical perspective". Selenium: 1–6. doi:10.1007/0-387-33827-6_1. ISBN 978-0-387-33826-2
- Williams, Rob (2006). Computer Systems Architecture: A Networking Approach. Prentice Hall. pp. 547–548. ISBN 978-0-321-34079-5
- Ohlendorf, H. M. (2003). Ecotoxicology of selenium. Handbook of ecotoxicology. Boca Raton: Lewis Publishers. pp. 466–491. ISBN 978-1-56670-546-2
- Mann, Jim; Truswell, A. Stewart (2002). Essentials of Human Nutrition (2nd ed.). Oxford University Press. ISBN 978-0-19-262756-8

4

Body Weight Management

Weight management is the process of maintaining a healthy body weight through the combination of various techniques. Weight management plays an important role in sports where an athlete has to maintain a certain body weight and deliver a good performance at the same time. Overweight, underweight, weight gain, weight loss, calorie restriction, meal replacement, etc. are a few terms associated with weight management which are discussed in detail in this chapter.

Weight management may be the most important focal area for nutrition and culinary specialists today. This is because the predictions for global overweight and obesity continue to rise, driving more opportunities. Weight loss is complex with so many variables that interfere with success, including dieting itself. Knowing the particulars of getting and keeping weight off provides the framework for well-designed, realistic, and satisfying diets, recipes, meals and menus.

Diets taken to the extreme become disordered eating. Anorexia and bulimia nervosa strike women and men of all ages. Eating more is not the answer. Working in tandem, nutrition and culinary professionals can team together at treatment facilities to ensure that even the smallest portions are rewarding.

The basic concept for weight management is simple and logical: the energy balance between intake and expenditure should be negative; in other words, energy intake should be decreased and activity increased. Yet changing habits is a great challenge and often community-based programmes facilitating such changes often fail to show long-term and clinically meaningful changes in weight status. The active participation and support of family members contributes to the success of any intervention, and ideally involvement of the whole family should be encouraged.

Weight management should start in childhood for overweight and obese individuals. Interventions with children should also be multicomponent and targeted to the individual, considering factors such as age and maturity. Interventions should include dietary modification, increased physical activity, decreased sedentary activity, family involvement, and behaviour modification.

The aim in young children, and in those where longitudinal growth is still occurring, is to stabilise weight gain such that the weight 'falls back' into normal ranges as the child grows. A stabilisation in weight gain, alongside normal increases in longitudinal growth, will lead to a decline in BMI back to normal over time. In older post-pubertal obese adolescents, a degree of weight loss may be required to achieve a 'normal' weight and BMI.

In essence, goals at reducing dietary intake and increasing physical activity should be individualised and based upon 'common sense' and not extreme recommendations, especially in young children. Here, the key is for the parents to try to change the environment of the child without the child really becoming aware of the parents' actions. Physical activity can be increased by encouragement into fun-based activities, whatever the situation – little equipment is required for children to become physically active. For example, younger children may only need a football to get more active, while older adolescents who need to train to achieve weight loss will be able to find useful 'equipment' to help them do this in any outdoor environment (e.g. sit-ups, press-ups, chin-ups and the like are all easily attainable in any outdoor parkland environment). Expensive gyms are not required, and even just increasing the amount of walking can often be beneficial in the first instance. Recommendations should be culturally sensitive and appropriate to the local resources.

Methods

Increase Intake of Protein, Especially at Breakfast

The satiating property of dietary protein is influenced by the time of protein consumption. Studies have shown that protein intake at breakfast has a greater satiety effect than later meal times. There are several explanations as to why this is the case. Firstly, protein has a greater thermogenic effect than carbohydrates and fat, which enables the body to burn more calories. Secondly, a high protein breakfast appears to slow gastric emptying, which attributes to the fact that protein appears to be the most satiating macronutrient. Finally, a high protein breakfast increases the activity of glucagon, which activates the pathways for glucose synthesis. One study showed that fat loss was approximately twice as much in the high-protein diet group than the moderate-protein diet group in overweight and obese individuals.

Plate Size

Using smaller plates helps to consume smaller portion sizes and this leads to the consumption of fewer calories. Studies have shown that portion size influences energy intake. People who are presented with larger portions do not report to have a higher level of satiety, which suggests that hunger and satiety signals are ignored when a large portion of food is placed in front of them. In particular, one study showed that participants consumed 31% less calories with the small portion sized of a 6-inch submarine sandwich compared with the large portion size of a 12-inch submarine sandwich. Increased portion sizes have occurred simultaneously with the increase in obesity rates; hence, large portion sizes can be one of the factors contributing to the current increase in body weight of the US. Evidence from a systematic review of 72 randomized controlled trials indicates that people consistently eat more food when offered larger portion, package, or tableware sizes rather than smaller size alternatives.

Eat More Soup

Soups have a significant satiety effect. Studies have demonstrated that compared to solid foods, soup ingestion decreases the amount of energy intake. Compared to having no soup, it has been shown that eating soup reduces total energy intake of a meal. When soup is consumed before a meal, a decrease of 20% of energy is consumed in the meal.

Choose Low-calorie Foods

A moderate decrease in caloric intake will lead to a slow weight loss, which may be more beneficial for long term weight management. For example, choosing a black coffee instead of a full fat latte will save calories that will add up in the long run. Low fat meats reduce the total amount of calories and cholesterol consumed. For example, traditional beef patties have 19.2% fat and 272 kcal per 100 g of meat. On the other hand, lean beef patties have 9.8%fat and 196 kcal.

Eating more Dairy can Aid in Fat Loss

Studies have shown that a diet high in dairy decreases total body fat. This occurs because a high amount of dietary calcium increases the amount of energy and fat excreted from the body. Studies have shown that saturated, monounsaturated and polyunsaturated fats all have a higher excretion rate with a high calcium intake. In these studies, a high calcium intake is considered 2300 mg and a low calcium intake is considered 700 mg. A possible explanation to this phenomenon is that high intakes of calcium cause calcium soap formation and/ or binding of bile acids in the intestine. Other studies specifically show that dairy sources of calcium demonstrate greater weight loss than supplemental calcium intake. This may be due to the other bioactive components present in milk, which may aid in metabolic efficiency and fat loss.

Incorporating more Vegetables into Meals

Fruits and vegetables have been shown to increase satiety and decrease hunger. These foods have a low energy density, which is mainly due to the high water content and partly due to the fiber content. The reduction of energy density has been shown to enhance satiety. The water adds weight, without adding calories and the fiber slows gastric emptying. Both of these factors contribute to the satiating effect of vegetables and fruits. Studies have also shown that fiber decreases hunger and also decreases total energy intake.

Fiber

Dietary fiber has been suggested to aid weight management by inducing satiety, decreasing absorption of macronutrients and promoting secretion of gut hormones. Dietary fiber consists of non-digestible carbohydrates and lignin, which are a structural component in plants. Fiber recommendations range from 10 – 13 grams/1000 calories, with slightly higher recommendations for men.

Due to the high volume or water content of fiber-rich foods, fiber displaces available calories and nutrients from the diet. Consumption of viscous fibers delays gastric emptying, which may cause an extended feeling of fullness. Satiety is also induced by increasing chewing, which limits food intake by promoting the secretion of saliva and gastric juice, resulting in an expansion of the stomach. In addition, hormone secretion is affected during fiber ingestion. Insulin response is reduced and cholecystokinin (CCK) in the small intestine is increased. Insulin regulates blood glucose levels while CCK adjusts gastric emptying, pancreatic secretion and gall bladder contraction. There is direct correlation between CCK and satiety after foods of different fiber contents are consumed. Fiber may have the added benefit of helping consumers decrease food intake throughout the day. However, results of trials examining this possibility have been conflicting. In general, large intakes of dietary fiber at breakfast are associated with less food intake at a lunch.

Resistant Starch

Resistant starch is a type of non-digestible, fermentable fiber that is resistant to amylase digestion in the small intestine, and is broken down to short-chain fatty acids by microflora in the large intestine. It is commonly found in cooked and cooled potatoes, green bananas, beans and legumes. Resistant starch dilutes energy density of food intake, has a bulking effect similar to non-fermentable fiber, and increases the expression of PYY and GLP-1 in the gut. The increase in gut hormones can affect long-term energy balance by affecting neuronal pathways in the brain as well as improved overall health of the intestines. Based on developing research, consumption of resistant starch can be an effective means of weight management.

Capsaicin

Clinical research on capsaicin has showed that consumption of the spice during breakfast can increase energy expenditure by 23% immediately after meal ingestion. Capsaicin, also known as hot pepper, is a primary ingredient in chilli peppers and red hot peppers. Hot peppers have been reported to induce thermogenesis at the cellular level.

As well, capsaicin induces satiety as a result of oral and gastro-intestinal contribution. Lower energy and fat intake were observed under short-term conditions;

however, the effect of the spice was reduced over prolonged exposure. Increased satiety was observed when oral contribution of capsaicin was measured in addition to the gastro-intestinal exposure, indicating the sensory effect of hot peppers plays a significant role.

Caffeine

Caffeine and black coffee have been associated with increased energy expenditure and subsequent weight loss. Caffeine belongs to a class of compounds called methylxanthines, and is present in coffee, tea, cocoa, chocolate and some cola drinks. Caffeine induces a thermogenic effect in the body by increasing sympathetic nervous system activity, which is an important regulator of energy expenditure.

Green Tea

Green tea has been associated with decreasing blood glucose, inhibiting hepatic and body fat accumulation, and stimulating thermogenesis due to the catechins that are present. Catechins are polyphenols that are a major component of green tea extract. Green tea has also been shown to increase energy expenditure and fat oxidation in humans, independent of the caffeine content(. In a human study conducted, 690 mg of catechins daily for 12 weeks reduced body fat, suggesting that green tea might be useful in the prevention of chronic disease, particularly obesity. Moreover, catechins in the brain play a major role in satiety.

Popular Diets

When assessing popular diets, a person's food preferences, lifestyle and medical conditions should be taken into account when choosing the correct diet. Adherence level to the diet is a bigger determinant of clinical benefits over the diet type itself. "Dieting" needs to be a lifestyle change rather than for a short term amount of time.

Weight Watchers

Weight Watchers offers a variety of dieting products and services to assist weight loss and maintenance by a calorie restricting method. Weight watchers promote healthy habits, a supportive environment, exercise and healthy food choices. A member to selects a goal weight that will result in a body mass index (BMI) generally accepted as healthy (18 – 24.9). Participants are encouraged to produce a rate of weight loss up to 2 pounds per week. Their food guide promotes food choices that not only reduce calories, but also meet nutritional recommendations. Exercise is also recommended for weight loss and is incorporated into their points system. They use a point system that incorporates calories, fat, and dietary fiber content of each food. People are given a certain number of points they are supposed to consume each day.

Strengths

- Their food guide promotes food choices that reduce calories, and also meet nutritional recommendations.
- They construct an activity plan along with nutritional guidelines to encourage exercise.
- They offer support and encouragement through weekly meetings.
- Is a slower weight loss than other more restrictive diets. This seems like a weakness, but most medical authorities recommend keeping weight loss at 1–2 pounds a week.

Limitations

- Can be quite expensive over time.

The Atkins Diet

The Atkins Diet involves the restriction of carbohydrates in one's diet causing the body's metabolism to switch from burning glucose as fuel to burning stored body fat, sending the body into a state of ketosis. Ketosis causes a person to get their energy from ketones, which also causes them to feel less hungry. Carbohydrate consumption must be <40 grams/day (= 2 slices of bread) for ketosis to occur.

Strengths

- Allowed to eat rich foods.
- When in ketosis, people feel less hungry and more satisfied.

Limitations

- Ketosis causes unusual breath odor and constipation.
- There is worry that the diet promotes heart disease and there is a potential loss of bone and it is not recommended for people with liver and kidney problems due to the high amounts of protein.
- The preferred source of energy for the brain is glucose, which is decreased in a low-carbohydrate diet.

GM Diet

The GM Diet was devised by the company General Motors to help its employees deal with weight gain due to sedentary work environment and achieve weight loss. The diet consists of low carbohydrates (they are primary fuel for anaerobic metabolism and strength training, a drastic depletion causes health risks) a 5–10g/kg body-weight which includes high fiber – nutrient dense starch whole foods for slow energy release and to increase satiety with fruits, tubers, vegetables etc., a moderate protein intake of 1.5–2.0g/kg body-weight along with 20-30g healthy fats daily (it supports natural hormonal and enzymatic functioning, improves insulin sensitivity, dilate blood vessels), drinking plenty of water and abstaining from alcohol (empty calories). The GM Diet works by burning off fat stored in body through creating a calorie deficit, with daily intake of required proportioned calorie amount, to ensure homeostatic balance.

Regular exercise is required to maintain the state of recovery from weight loss management. If resistance training is employed to maintain muscle mass for better glucose-disposal and glucose-control capability, a 12 to 48 hours of rest between sessions is a required time for the muscles to recover depending on intensity of exercise or training load. A change in hormone levels occurs in case of drastic dietary changes, like leptin - a satiety hormone, made by fat cells showed declination in levels, its function is to regulate energy balance by inhibiting hunger and at the same time, there is also a rise in levels of ghrelin - a hormone secreted in the gastrointestinal tract when a person's stomach is empty and informs one they are hungry. Changes in production of these hormones along with other satiating hormones in extreme weight loss managements showed suppressed resting metabolic rate (RMR) which resulted many subjects regaining much of the lost weight.

Ornish Diet

The Ornish Diet is a fat restricting diet (less than 10% of calories from fat) focusing on eating high amounts of fiber, and following a low-fat vegetarian diet. The Ornish diet recommends combining the diet with exercise that allows the body's fat burning mechanism to work most effectively. The philosophy is focused less on restricting calories but by watching the ones consumed, by recommending foods that can be eaten all the time, some of the time and none of the time.

Foods that can be eaten whenever hungry until one is full are:

- Beans and legumes, fruits, grains and vegetables.

Foods eaten in moderation are:

- Nonfat dairy products – skim milk, nonfat yogurt, nonfat cheese, nonfat sour cream and egg whites.

Foods to avoid

- Meats of all kinds – if can't give up, only eat minimally.
- Oils and oil-containing products (margarine and most salad dressings).
- Avocados, olives, nuts and seeds, dairy products (other than non-fat ones).
- Simple sugar and simple sugar derivatives (honey, molassess, corn syrup, and high-fructose syrup).

- Alcohol.
- Anything commercially prepared that has more than 2 grams of fat per serving.

Suggests eating a lot of little meals because this diet makes people feel hungry more often, which will help them feel full faster and eat more food without increasing the number of calories.

Strengths

- Does not restrict calories.
- Doesn't slow down metabolism.
- Recommends regular exercise, yoga and meditation along with the diet.
- Has been associated with a reversal of coronary blockage.

Weakness

- Very restrictive.
- People will feel hungrier and need to eat more food (but less calories).

Overweight

Obesity is when a person is carrying too much body fat for their height and sex. A person is considered obese if they have a body mass index (BMI) of 30 or greater.

Today's way of life is less physically active than it used to be. People travel on buses and cars, rather than walking, and many people work in offices, where they are sitting still for most of the day. This means that the calories they eat are not getting burnt off as energy. Instead, the extra calories are stored as fat.

Over time, eating excess calories leads to weight gain. Without lifestyle changes to increase the amount of physical activity done on a daily basis, or reduce the amount of calories consumed, people can become obese.

Obesity can be measured in different ways. An easy way is to simply step on the scales and compare your actual weight with your ideal weight.

The most widely used way to measure your weight is to calculate your body mass index (BMI). This is your weight in kilograms divided by your height in metres squared.

- If your BMI is between 25 and 29.9, you are over the ideal weight for your height (overweight).
- If your BMI is between 30 and 39.9, you are obese.

- If your BMI is over 40, you are very obese (known as 'morbidly obese').

Classification

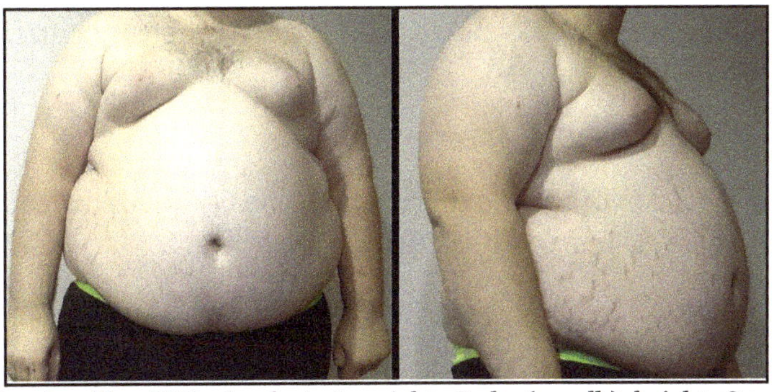

A "super obese" male with a BMI of 53 kg/m^2: weight 182 kg (400 lb), height 185 cm (6 ft 1 in). He presents with stretch marks and enlarged breasts.

BMI (kg/m^2)		Classification
from	up to	
	18.5	underweight
18.5	25.0	normal weight
25.0	30.0	overweight
30.0	35.0	class I obesity
35.0	40.0	class II obesity
40.0		class III obesity

Obesity is a medical condition in which excess body fat has accumulated to the extent that it may have an adverse effect on health. It is defined by body mass index (BMI) and further evaluated in terms of fat distribution via the waist–hip ratio and total cardiovascular risk factors. BMI is closely related to both percentage body fat and total body fat. In children, a healthy weight varies with age and sex. Obesity in children and adolescents is defined not as an absolute number but in relation to a historical normal group, such that obesity is a BMI greater than the 95th percentile. The reference data on which these percentiles were based date from 1963 to 1994, and thus have not been affected by the recent increases in weight. BMI is defined as the subject's weight divided by the square of their height and is calculated as follows.

$$\mathrm{BMI} = \frac{m}{h^2},$$

where m and h are the subject's weight and height respectively.

BMI is usually expressed in kilograms per square metre, resulting when weight is measured in kilograms and height in metres. To convert from pounds per square inch multiply by 703 (kg/m^2)/(lb/sq in).

The most commonly used definitions, established by the World Health Organization (WHO) in 1997 and published in 2000, provide the values listed in the table.

Some modifications to the WHO definitions have been made by particular organizations. The surgical literature breaks down class II and III obesity into further categories whose exact values are still disputed.

- Any BMI ≥ 35 or 40 kg/m² is *severe obesity.*
- A BMI of ≥ 35 kg/m² and experiencing obesity-related health conditions or ≥40–44.9 kg/m² is *morbid obesity.*
- A BMI of ≥ 45 or 50 kg/m² is *super obesity.*

As Asian populations develop negative health consequences at a lower BMI than Caucasians, some nations have redefined obesity; Japan have defined obesity as any BMI greater than 25 kg/m² while China uses a BMI of greater than 28 kg/m².

Effects on Health

Excessive body weight is associated with various diseases and conditions, particularly cardiovascular diseases, diabetes mellitus type 2, obstructive sleep apnea, certain types of cancer, osteoarthritis, and asthma. As a result, obesity has been found to reduce life expectancy.

Mortality

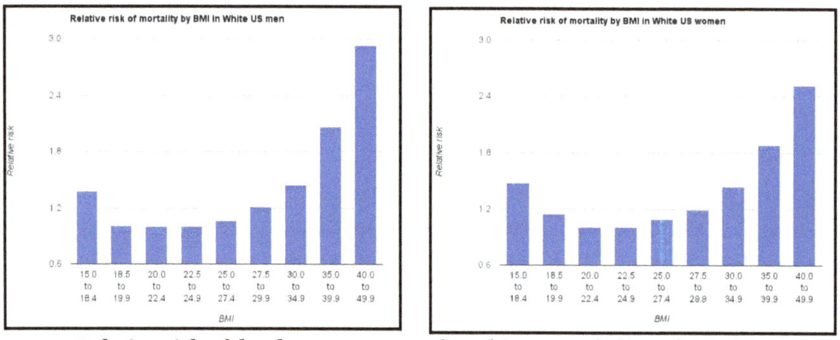

Relative risk of death over 10 years for white men (left) and women (right) who have never smoked.

Obesity is one of the leading preventable causes of death worldwide. A number of reviews have found that mortality risk is lowest at a BMI of 20–25 kg/m² in non-smokers and at 24–27 kg/m² in current smokers, with risk increasing along with changes in either direction. This appears to apply in at least four continents. In contrast, a 2013 review found that grade 1 obesity (BMI 30–35) was not associated with higher mortality than normal weight, and that overweight (BMI 25–30) was associated with "lower" mortality than was normal weight (BMI 18.5–25). Other evidence suggests that the association of BMI and waist circumference with mortality is U- or J-shaped, while the association between waist-to-hip ratio and waist-to-height ratio with mortality is more positive. In Asians the risk of negative health effects begins to increase between 22–25 kg/m². A BMI above 32 kg/m² has been associated with a doubled mortality rate among women over a 16-year period. In the United States, obesity is estimated to cause 111,909 to 365,000 deaths per year, while 1 million (7.7%) of deaths in Europe are attributed to excess weight. On average, obesity reduces life expectancy by six to seven years, a BMI of 30–35 kg/m² reduces life expectancy by two to four years, while severe obesity (BMI > 40 kg/m²) reduces life expectancy by ten years.

Morbidity

Obesity increases the risk of many physical and mental conditions. These comorbidities are most commonly shown in metabolic syndrome, a combination of medical disorders which includes: diabetes mellitus type 2, high blood pressure, high blood cholesterol, and high triglyceride levels.

Complications are either directly caused by obesity or indirectly related through mechanisms sharing a common cause such as a poor diet or a sedentary lifestyle. The strength of the link between obesity and specific conditions varies. One of the strongest is the link with type 2 diabetes. Excess body fat underlies 64% of cases of diabetes in men and 77% of cases in women.

Health consequences fall into two broad categories: those attributable to the effects of increased fat mass (such as osteoarthritis, obstructive sleep apnea, social stigmatization) and those due to the increased number of fat cells (diabetes, cancer, cardiovascular disease, non-alcoholic fatty liver disease). Increases in body fat alter the body's response to insulin, potentially leading to insulin resistance. Increased fat also creates a proinflammatory state, and a prothrombotic state.

Medical field	Condition	Medical field	Condition
Cardiology	• coronary heart disease: angina and myocardial infarction • congestive heart failure • high blood pressure • abnormal cholesterol levels • deep vein thrombosis and pulmonary embolism	Dermatology	• stretch marks • acanthosis nigricans • lymphedema • cellulitis • hirsutism • intertrigo
Endocrinology and Reproductive medicine	• diabetes mellitus • polycystic ovarian syndrome • menstrual disorders • infertility • complications during pregnancy • birth defects • intrauterine fetal death	Gastroenterology	• gastroesophageal reflux disease • fatty liver disease • cholelithiasis (gallstones)

Neurology	• stroke • meralgia paresthetica • migraines • carpal tunnel syndrome • dementia • idiopathic intracranial hypertension • multiple sclerosis	Oncology	• esophageal • colorectal • pancreatic • gallbladder • endometrial • kidney • Leukemia • Hepatocellular carcinoma • malignant melanoma
Psychiatry	• depression in women • social stigmatization	Respirology	• obstructive sleep apnea • obesity hypoventilation syndrome • asthma • increased complications during general anaesthesia
Rheumatology and Orthopedics	• gout • poor mobility • osteoarthritis • low back pain	Urology and Nephrology	• erectile dysfunction • urinary incontinence • chronic renal failure • hypogonadism • buried penis

Survival Paradox

Although the negative health consequences of obesity in the general population are well supported by the available evidence, health outcomes in certain subgroups seem to be improved at an increased BMI, a phenomenon known as the obesity survival paradox. The paradox was first described in 1999 in overweight and obese people undergoing hemodialysis, and has subsequently been found in those with heart failure and peripheral artery disease (PAD).

In people with heart failure, those with a BMI between 30.0 and 34.9 had lower mortality than those with a normal weight. This has been attributed to the fact that people often lose weight as they become progressively more ill. Similar findings have been made in other types of heart disease. People with class I obesity and heart disease do not have greater rates of further heart problems than people of normal weight who also have heart disease. In people with greater degrees of obesity, however, the risk of further cardiovascular events is increased. Even after cardiac bypass surgery, no increase in mortality is seen in the overweight and obese. One study found that the improved survival could be explained by the more aggressive treatment obese people receive after a cardiac event. Another found that if one takes into account chronic obstructive pulmonary disease (COPD) in those with PAD, the benefit of obesity no longer exists.

Causes

At an individual level, a combination of excessive food energy intake and a lack of physical activity is thought to explain most cases of obesity. A limited number of cases are due primarily to genetics, medical reasons, or psychiatric illness. In contrast, increasing rates of obesity at a societal level are felt to be due to an easily accessible and palatable diet, increased reliance on cars, and mechanized manufacturing.

A 2006 review identified ten other possible contributors to the recent increase of obesity: (1) insufficient sleep, (2) endocrine disruptors (environmental pollutants that interfere with lipid metabolism), (3) decreased variability in ambient temperature, (4) decreased rates of smoking, because smoking suppresses appetite, (5) increased use of medications that can cause weight gain (e.g., atypical antipsychotics), (6) proportional increases in ethnic and age groups that tend to be heavier, (7) pregnancy at a later age (which may cause susceptibility to obesity in children), (8) epigenetic risk factors passed on generationally, (9) natural selection for higher BMI, and (10) assortative mating leading to increased concentration of obesity risk factors (this would increase the number of obese people by increasing population variance in weight). While there is evidence supporting the influence of these mechanisms on the increased prevalence of obesity, the evidence is still inconclusive, and the authors state that these are probably less influential than the ones discussed in the previous paragraph.

Diet

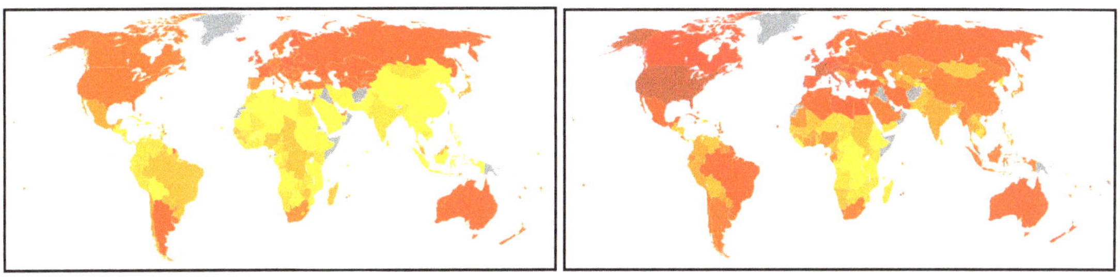

1961 2001–03

Map of dietary energy availability per person per day in 1961 (left) and 2001–2003 (right) Calories per person per day (kilojoules per person per day)

- no data
- <1,600 (<6,700)
- 1,600–1,800 (6,700–7,500)
- 1,800–2,000 (7,500–8,400)
- 2,000–2,200 (8,400–9,200)
- 2,200–2,400 (9,200–10,000)
- 2,400–2,600 (10,000–10,900)
- 2,600–2,800 (10,900–11,700)
- 2,800–3,000 (11,700–12,600)
- 3,000–3,200 (12,600–13,400)
- 3,200–3,400 (13,400–14,200)
- 3,400–3,600 (14,200–15,100)
- >3,600 (>15,100)

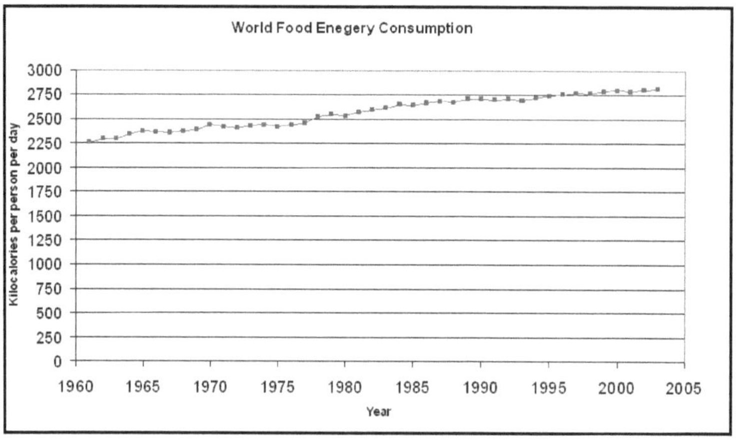

Average per capita energy consumption of the world from 1961 to 2002

A 2016 review supported excess food as the primary factor. Dietary energy supply per capita varies markedly between different regions and countries. It has also changed significantly over time. From the early 1970s to the late 1990s the average food energy available per person per day (the amount of food bought) increased in all parts of the world except Eastern Europe. The United States had the highest availability with 3,654 calories (15,290 kJ) per person in 1996. This increased further in 2003 to 3,754 calories (15,710 kJ). During the late 1990s Europeans had 3,394 calories (14,200 kJ) per person, in the developing areas of Asia there were 2,648 calories (11,080 kJ) per person, and in sub-Saharan Africa people had 2,176 calories (9,100 kJ) per person. Total food energy consumption has been found to be related to obesity.

The widespread availability of nutritional guidelines has done little to address the problems of overeating and poor dietary choice. From 1971 to 2000, obesity rates in the United States increased from 14.5% to 30.9%. During the same period, an increase occurred in the average amount of food energy consumed. For women, the average increase was 335 calories (1,400 kJ) per day (1,542 calories (6,450 kJ) in 1971 and 1,877 calories (7,850 kJ) in 2004), while for men the average increase was 168 calories (700 kJ) per day (2,450 calories (10,300 kJ) in 1971 and 2,618 calories (10,950 kJ) in 2004). Most of this extra food energy came from an increase in carbohydrate consumption rather than fat consumption. The primary sources of these extra carbohydrates are sweetened beverages, which now account for almost 25 percent of daily food energy in young adults in America, and potato chips. Consumption of sweetened drinks such as soft drinks, fruit drinks, iced tea, and energy and vitamin water drinks is believed to be contributing to the rising rates of obesity and to an increased risk of metabolic syndrome and type 2 diabetes. Vitamin D deficiency is related to diseases associated with obesity.

As societies become increasingly reliant on energy-dense, big-portions, and fast-food meals, the association between fast-food consumption and obesity becomes more concerning. In the United States consumption of fast-food meals tripled and food energy intake from these meals quadrupled between 1977 and 1995.

Agricultural policy and techniques in the United States and Europe have led to lower food prices. In the United States, subsidization of corn, soy, wheat, and rice through the U.S. farm bill has made the main sources of processed food cheap compared to fruits and vegetables. Calorie count laws and nutrition facts labels attempt to steer people toward making healthier food choices, including awareness of how much food energy is being consumed.

Obese people consistently under-report their food consumption as compared to people of normal weight. This is supported both by tests of people carried out in a calorimeter room and by direct observation.

Sedentary Lifestyle

A sedentary lifestyle plays a significant role in obesity. Worldwide there has been a large shift towards less physically demanding work, and currently at least 30% of the world's population gets insufficient exercise. This is primarily due to increasing use of mechanized transportation and a greater prevalence of labor-saving technology in the home. In children, there appear to be declines in levels of physical activity due to less walking and physical education. World trends in active leisure time physical activity are less clear. The World Health Organization indicates people worldwide are taking up less active recreational pursuits, while a study from Finland found an increase and a study from the United States found leisure-time physical activity has not changed significantly. A 2011 review of physical activity in children found that it may not be a significant contributor.

In both children and adults, there is an association between television viewing time and the risk of obesity. A review found 63 of 73 studies (86%) showed an increased rate of childhood obesity with increased media exposure, with rates increasing proportionally to time spent watching television.

Genetics

Like many other medical conditions, obesity is the result of an interplay between genetic and environmental factors. Polymorphisms in various genes controlling appetite and metabolism predispose to obesity when sufficient food energy is present. As of 2006, more than 41 of these sites on the human genome have been linked to the development of obesity when a favorable environment is present. People with two copies of the FTO gene (fat mass and obesity associated gene) have been found on average to weigh 3–4 kg more and have a 1.67-fold greater risk of obesity compared with those without the risk allele. The differences in BMI between people that are due to genetics varies depending on the population examined from 6% to 85%.

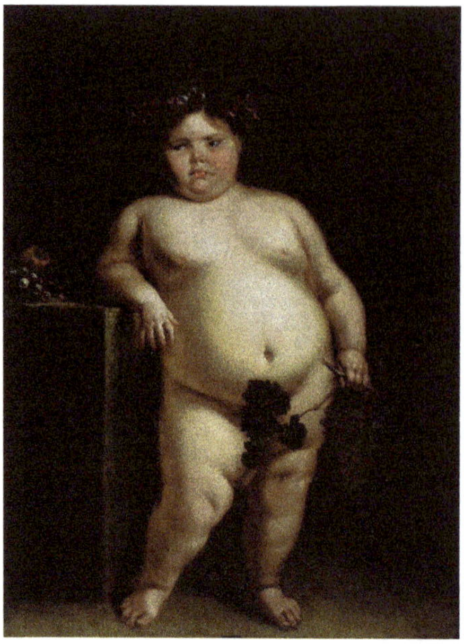

A painting of a girl presumed to have Prader–Willi syndrome.

Obesity is a major feature in several syndromes, such as Prader–Willi syndrome, Bardet–Biedl syndrome, Cohen syndrome, and MOMO syndrome. (The term "non-syndromic obesity" is sometimes used to exclude these conditions.) In people with early-onset severe obesity (defined by an onset before 10 years of age and body mass index over three standard deviations above normal), 7% harbor a single point DNA mutation.

Studies that have focused on inheritance patterns rather than on specific genes have found that 80% of the offspring of two obese parents were also obese, in contrast to less than 10% of the offspring of two parents who were of normal weight. Different people exposed to the same environment have different risks of obesity due to their underlying genetics.

The thrifty gene hypothesis postulates that, due to dietary scarcity during human evolution, people are prone to obesity. Their ability to take advantage of rare periods of abundance by storing energy as fat would be advantageous during times of varying food availability, and individuals with greater adipose reserves would be more likely to survive famine. This tendency to store fat, however, would be maladaptive in societies with stable food supplies. This theory has received various criticisms, and other evolutionarily-based theories such as the drifty gene hypothesis and the thrifty phenotype hypothesis have also been proposed.

Other Illnesses

Certain physical and mental illnesses and the pharmaceutical substances used to treat them can increase risk of obesity. Medical illnesses that increase obesity risk include several rare genetic syndromes (listed above) as well as some congenital or acquired conditions: hypothyroidism, Cushing's syndrome, growth hormone deficiency, and the eating disorders: binge eating disorder and night eating syndrome. However, obesity is not regarded as a psychiatric disorder, and therefore is not listed in the DSM-IVR as a psychiatric illness. The risk of overweight and obesity is higher in patients with psychiatric disorders than in persons without psychiatric disorders.

Certain medications may cause weight gain or changes in body composition; these include insulin, sulfonylureas, thiazolidinediones, atypical antipsychotics, antidepressants, steroids, certain anticonvulsants (phenytoin and valproate), pizotifen, and some forms of hormonal contraception.

Social Determinants

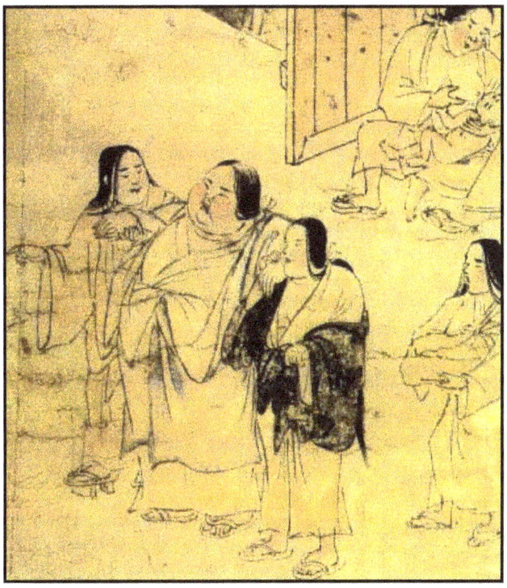

The disease scroll depicts a woman moneylender with obesity, considered a disease of the rich.

While genetic influences are important to understanding obesity, they cannot explain the current dramatic increase seen within specific countries or globally. Though it is accepted that energy consumption in excess of energy expenditure leads to obesity on an individual basis, the cause of the shifts in these two factors on the societal scale is much debated. There are a number of theories as to the cause but most believe it is a combination of various factors.

The correlation between social class and BMI varies globally. A review in 1989 found that in developed countries women of a high social class were less likely to be obese. No significant differences were seen among men of different social classes. In the developing world, women, men, and children from high social classes had greater rates of obesity. An update of this review carried out in 2007 found the same relationships, but they were weaker. The decrease in strength of correlation was felt to be due to the effects of globalization. Among developed countries, levels of adult obesity, and percentage of teenage children who are overweight, are correlated with income inequality. A similar relationship is seen among US states: more adults, even in higher social classes, are obese in more unequal states.

Many explanations have been put forth for associations between BMI and social class. It is thought that in developed countries, the wealthy are able to afford more nutritious food, they are under greater social pressure to remain slim, and have more opportunities along with greater expectations for physical fitness. In undeveloped countries the ability to afford food, high energy expenditure with physical labor, and cultural values favoring a larger body size are believed to contribute to the observed patterns. Attitudes toward body weight held by people in one's life may also play a role in obesity. A correlation in BMI changes over time has been found among friends, siblings, and spouses. Stress and perceived low social status appear to increase risk of obesity.

Smoking has a significant effect on an individual's weight. Those who quit smoking gain an average of 4.4 kilograms (9.7 lb) for men and 5.0 kilograms (11.0 lb) for women over ten years. However, changing rates of smoking have had little effect on the overall rates of obesity.

In the United States the number of children a person has is related to their risk of obesity. A woman's risk increases by 7% per child, while a man's risk increases by 4% per child. This could be partly explained by the fact that having dependent children decreases physical activity in Western parents.

In the developing world urbanization is playing a role in increasing rate of obesity. In China overall rates of obesity are below 5%; however, in some cities rates of obesity are greater than 20%.

Malnutrition in early life is believed to play a role in the rising rates of obesity in the developing world. Endocrine changes that occur during periods of malnutrition may promote the storage of fat once more food energy becomes available.

Consistent with cognitive epidemiological data, numerous studies confirm that obesity is associated with cognitive deficits. Whether obesity causes cognitive deficits, or vice versa is unclear at present.

Gut Bacteria

The study of the effect of infectious agents on metabolism is still in its early stages. Gut flora has been shown to differ between lean and obese humans. There is an indication that gut flora in obese and lean individuals can affect the metabolic potential. This apparent alteration of the metabolic potential is believed to confer a greater capacity to harvest energy contributing to obesity. Whether these differences are the direct cause or the result of obesity has yet to be determined unequivocally. The use of antibiotics among children has also been associated with obesity later in life.

An association between viruses and obesity has been found in humans and several different animal species. The amount that these associations may have contributed to the rising rate of obesity is yet to be determined.

Management

The main treatment for obesity consists of dieting and physical exercise. Diet programs may produce weight loss over the short term, but maintaining this weight loss is frequently difficult and often requires making exercise and a lower food energy diet a permanent part of a person's lifestyle.

In the short-term low carbohydrate diets appear better than low fat diets for weight loss. In the long term; however, all types of low-carbohydrate and low-fat diets appear equally beneficial. A 2014 review found that the heart disease and diabetes risks associated with different diets appear to be similar. Promotion of the Mediterranean diets among the obese may lower the risk of heart disease. Decreased intake of sweet drinks is also related to weight-loss. Success rates of long-term weight loss maintenance with lifestyle changes are low, ranging from 2–20%. Dietary and lifestyle changes are effective in limiting excessive weight gain in pregnancy and improve outcomes for both the mother and the child. Intensive behavioral counseling is recommended in those who are both obese and have other risk factors for heart disease.

Five medications have evidence for long-term use orlistat, lorcaserin, liraglutide, phentermine–topiramate, and naltrexone–bupropion. They result in weight loss after one year ranged from 3.0 to 6.7 kg (6.6-14.8 lbs) over placebo. Orlistat, liraglutide, and naltrexone–bupropion are available in both the United States and Europe, whereas lorcaserin and phentermine–topiramate are available only in the United States. European regulatory authorities rejected the latter two drugs in part because of associations of heart valve problems with lorcaserin and more general heart and blood vessel problems with phentermine–topiramate. Orlistat use is associated with high rates of gastrointestinal side effects and concerns have been raised about negative effects on the kidneys. There is no information on how these drugs affect longer-term complications of obesity such as cardiovascular disease or death.

The most effective treatment for obesity is bariatric surgery. The types of procedures include laparoscopic adjustable gastric banding, Roux-en-Y gastric bypass, vertical-sleeve gastrectomy, and biliopancreatic diversion. Surgery for severe obesity is associated with long-term weight loss, improvement in obesity-related conditions, and decreased overall mortality. One study found a weight loss of between 14% and 25% (depending on the type of procedure performed) at 10 years, and a 29% reduction in all cause mortality when compared to standard weight loss measures. Complications occur in about 17% of cases and reoperation is needed in 7% of cases. Due to its cost and risks, researchers are searching for other effective yet less invasive treatments including devices that occupy space in the stomach.

Epidemiology

In earlier historical periods obesity was rare, and achievable only by a small elite, although already recognised as a problem for health. But as prosperity increased in the Early Modern period, it affected increasingly larger groups of the population.

In 1997 the WHO formally recognized obesity as a global epidemic. As of 2008 the WHO estimates that at least 500 million adults (greater than 10%) are obese, with higher rates among women than men. The percentage of adults affected in the United States as of 2015-2016 is about 39.6% overall (37.9% of males and 41.1% of females).

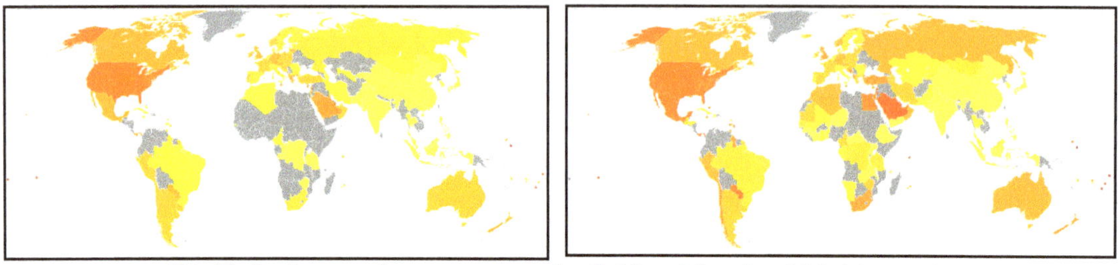

World obesity prevalence among males (left) and females (right) in 2008.

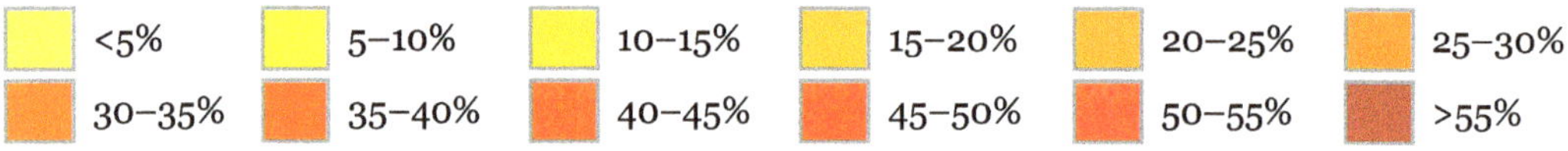

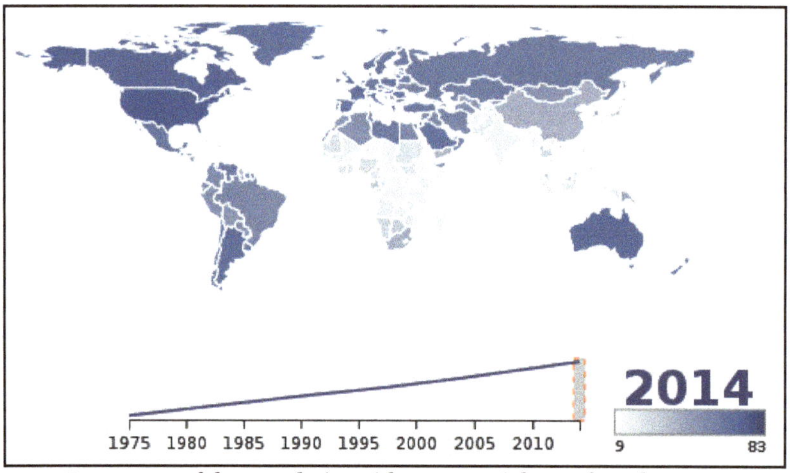

Percentage of the population either overweight or obese by year.

The rate of obesity also increases with age at least up to 50 or 60 years old and severe obesity in the United States, Australia, and Canada is increasing faster than the overall rate of obesity.

Once considered a problem only of high-income countries, obesity rates are rising worldwide and affecting both the developed and developing world. These increases have been felt most dramatically in urban settings. The only remaining region of the world where obesity is not common is sub-Saharan Africa.

Childhood Obesity

The healthy BMI range varies with the age and sex of the child. Obesity in children and adolescents is defined as a BMI greater than the 95th percentile. The reference data that these percentiles are based on is from 1963 to 1994 and thus has not been affected by the recent increases in rates of obesity. Childhood obesity has reached epidemic proportions in the 21st century, with rising rates in both the developed and the developing world. Rates of obesity in Canadian boys have increased from 11% in the 1980s to over 30% in the 1990s, while during this same time period rates increased from 4 to 14% in Brazilian children.

As with obesity in adults, many factors contribute to the rising rates of childhood obesity. Changing diet and decreasing physical activity are believed to be the two most important causes for the recent increase in the incidence of child obesity. Because childhood obesity often persists into adulthood and is associated with numerous chronic illnesses, children who are obese are often tested for hypertension, diabetes, hyperlipidemia, and fatty liver. Treatments used in children are primarily lifestyle interventions and behavioral techniques, although efforts to increase activity in children have had little success. In the United States, medications are not FDA approved for use in this age group. Multi-component behaviour change interventions that include changes to dietary and physical activity may reduce BMI in the short term in children aged 6 to 11 years, although the benefits are small and quality of evidence is low.

Underweight

An underweight person is an individual whose body mass index or BMI is under 18.5, or has a weight which is around 15 to 20 percent below the normal as determined by the age and height group to which the person belongs. Being underweight is generally considered a sign of ill-health and be symptomatic of some underlying disease. The contributing factors to this condition are genetics, substance abuse, a high metabolism, eating disorder or physical or mental illness. Some medical conditions associated with being underweight are hyperthyroidism, diabetes, cancer and tuberculosis. Problems associated with the liver or the gastrointestine may also induce loss of weight, primarily due to the inability to absorb nutrients in adequate quantities. It can also be caused due to the intake of a diet that does not consist of the necessary nutrients or if the individual is over worked. The long term effects of being underweight are significant. People who are underweight are more prone to osteoporosis, anemia, amenorrhea, infertility and even complications during pregnancy.

Considering the consequences of this condition, it is vital to manage a healthy body weight for good health and welfare. A way to achieve this is by taking a high calorie intake, exercising regularly or by taking medication that suppresses the factors contributing to the loss of weight. Such drugs may include antidepressants, antipsychotics and supplements.

Signs of Being Underweight

If you are underweight, you may notice certain signs on your body. But some symptoms commonly associated with thinness may have other causes. For example, do veiny arms mean you're underweight? Some people who are very thin complain about veiny arms. Medical experts say that being too thin can cause dry, thin skin which might make veins look more obvious. But bodybuilders have veiny arms, as well. So veiny arms, alone, aren't necessarily an indicator that you are too thin.

Other people complain about joints that look too large. If you are underweight and carry very little muscle mass, your bones and your joints may appear more prominent. But again, having large bones or a more noticeable joint doesn't mean that you are definitely underweight.

Other symptoms of being underweight may include:

- Fragile bones,
- Irregular menstrual periods or problems getting pregnant,
- Hair loss,
- Weak immune system,
- Dizziness or fatigue from anemia,
- Poor growth and development, especially in children who are underweight.

Causes

A person may be underweight due to genetics, metabolism, drug use, lack of food (frequently due to poverty), eating disorder, or illness (both physical and mental).

Being underweight is associated with certain medical conditions, including diabetes, hyperthyroidism, cancer, or tuberculosis. People with gastrointestinal or liver problems may be unable to absorb nutrients adequately. People with certain eating disorders can also be underweight due to lack of nutrients/over exercise.

Problems

Underweight might be secondary to or symptomatic of an underlying disease. Unexplained weight loss may require professional medical diagnosis.

Underweight can also be a primary causative condition. Severely underweight individuals may have poor physical stamina and a weak immune system, leaving them open to infection. "Underweight status and micronutrient deficiencies also cause decreases in immune and non-immune host defenses, and should be classified as underlying causes of death if followed by infectious diseases that are the terminal associated causes." People who are malnutrative underweight raise special concerns, as not only gross caloric intake may be inadequate, but also intake and absorption of other vital nutrients, especially essential amino acids and micro-nutrients such as vitamins and minerals.

In women, being severely underweight as a result of an eating disorder, or due to excessive strenuous exercise can result in amenorrhea (absence of menstruation), infertility and, if gestational weight gain is too low, possible complications during pregnancy. Malnourishment can also cause anemia and hair loss.

Being underweight is an established risk factor for osteoporosis, even for young people. This is seen in individuals suffering from the female athlete triad, when disordered eating or excessive exercise cause amenorrhea, hormone changes during an ovulation leads to loss of bone mineral density. After the occurrence of first spontaneous fractures the damage is often already irreversible.

Although being underweight has been reported to increase mortality at rates comparable to that seen in morbidly obese people, the effect is much less drastic when restricted to non-smokers with no history of disease, suggesting that smoking and disease-related weight loss are the leading causes of the observed effect.

Treatment

Diet

Underweight individuals may be advised to gain weight by increasing calorie intake. This can be done by eating a sufficient volume of sufficiently calorie-dense foods. Body weight may also be increased through the consumption of liquid nutritional supplements. Other nutritional supplements may be recommended for individuals with insufficient vitamin or mineral intake.

Exercise

Another way for underweight people to gain weight is by exercising. Muscle hypertrophy increases body mass. Weight lifting exercises are effective in helping to improve muscle tone as well as helping with weight gain. Weight lifting has also been shown to improve bone mineral density, for which underweight people have an increased risk of deficiency.

Exercise itself is catabolic, which results in a brief reduction in mass. The gain in weight that can result of it comes from the anabolic overcompensation when the body recovers and overcompensates via muscle hypertrophy. This can happen by an increase in the muscle proteins, or through enhanced storage of glycogen in muscles. Exercise can help stimulate a person's appetite if they are not inclined to eat.

Appetite Stimulants

Certain drugs may increase appetite either as their primary effect or as a side effect. Antidepressants, such as mirtazapine or amitriptyline, and antipsychotics, particularly chlorpromazine and haloperidol, as well as tetrahydrocannabinol (found in cannabis), all present an increase in appetite as a side effect. In states where it is approved, medicinal cannabis may be prescribed for severe appetite loss, such as that caused by cancer, AIDS, or severe levels of persistent anxiety. Other drugs or supplements which may increase appetite include antihistamines (such as diphenhydramine, promethazine or cyproheptadine), and B vitamin supplements (such as vitamin B12 and vitamin B-complex).

Weight Gain

Weight gain refers to an increase in body weight owing to an increase in fat deposits, muscle mass or bodily fluids such as water. While weight gain may be a requirement for individuals with lower than normal BMI, it can be highly undesirable for people who are overweight. In some cases, gaining weight can be symptomatic of a serious medical condition. The contribution of eating to weight gain varies depending on the energy calorie density of foods, amount of water and salt intake, exercise regimen followed, age, stress level and even the time of day the food is eaten. In modern sedentary lifestyles with high food intake, obesity is a growing concern. In a recent study of the American population, it was found that more than half the population of the United States is overweight or obese.

Increased food consumption and wrong lifestyle choices play the most significant role in weight gain, Inadequate sleep and excessive stress can lead to increased appetite and also reduce energy expenditure, while certain psychiatric medications can also cause weight gain. Certain medical conditions such as hypothyroidism, insulinoma, Cushing's syndrome, Bardet-Beidl syndrome, Cohen syndrome, etc. can contribute to weight gain. Excess weight is seen as unacceptable in modern society. As such, many weight loss regimens, physical fitness products and surgeries have risen in popularity. Further, the stigma associated with weight gain can have an adverse effect on the mental state if the modern youth, especially young women. It is in the interest of all, therefore, to promote a positive image and respect for the body and also adhere to regular exercising and proper diet to lead a happy healthy life.

Causes of Weight Gain

The number of overweight and obese people steadily increases each year. Weight gain is now a major worldwide problem. The main problem with weight gain is its negative effect on a person's health. In order to find the best solution to this problem, you need to be aware of the many different causes of weight gain. Take note that it is not always connected to your food intake and physical activity level. There is a possibility that the weight gain you are experiencing is due to an underlying medical condition or any other reason.

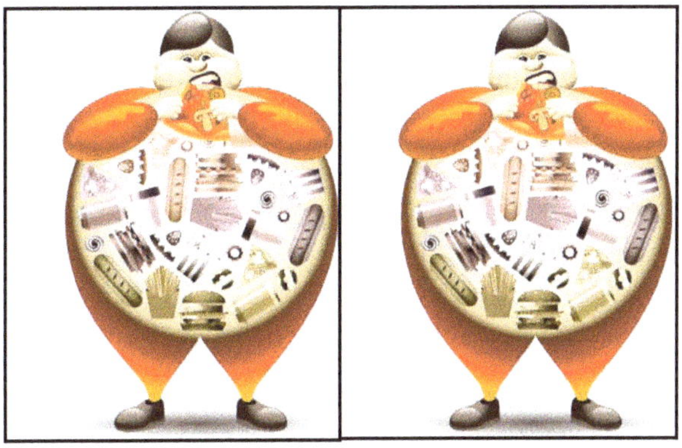

Unintentional weight gain is simply when you gain weight without trying to do so. On the other hand, intentional weight gain is when you gain weight because you eat more like when you're trying to gain muscle mass or increase weight to reach your ideal weight. Here are the most common causes of weight gain:

Digestive Causes:

> There are many reasons why poor digestion can cause weight gain. If the body is having problems breaking down food, eliminating toxins and absorbing nutrients, the metabolism slows down leading to weight gain. People with digestive problems don't absorb essential nutrients sufficiently. This includes iron, magnesium, B-vitamins and other nutrients that play a vital role in the process of burning calories. The common result is fatigue and the accumulation of excess body fat. Toxic build-ups can also cause puffiness, sluggishness and make it difficult to lose weight. It can also promote the retention of excess water in the body.

Endocrine System Problems:

> There is a very close connection between hormones and weight gain. Hormonal imbalances can cause weight gain. There are a number of endocrine disorders that can cause unintentional weight gain such as hypothyroidism and Cushing's syndrome. Weight gain is the result when the body is not able to utilize the energy put into it through food consumption. Hormones play a very important role in metabolizing food for energy and appetite.

Urinary Problems:

> One of the most common causes of weight gain is carrying excess fluids or water retention. This usually occurs when there is something with the body's ability to eliminate excess fluids or there are disorders related to the urinary system. If this is the case then medical treatment is necessary to treat the problem and get rid of the water retention and excess weight.

Medications:

Certain medications can also cause weight gain and make weight loss almost impossible. This includes some prescription drugs for treating mood disorders, depression, migraines, high blood pressure and diabetes. Hormone replacement therapy, steroids and oral contraceptives may also cause weight gain in some people. These drugs work differently in causing weight gain. It may be from increasing the appetite, altering the body's fat storage process or insulin level changes.

Lack of Sleep:

The body needs quality sleep for optimal functioning. When you don't get enough sleep, the body experiences physiological stress which alters the way it stores fat and at the same time slows down metabolism. Also, when you're tired due to lack of sleep, the body has a harder time dealing with stress. This often causes emotional eating or turning to food for comfort or as a coping mechanism. You need around 6-8 hours of sleep every night.

Age:

One of the most common causes of weight gain is aging. As you get older, your metabolism slows down and the body burns fewer calories daily. This means that you should be eating less as you get older. You should also perform more physical activities like exercise in order to prevent weight gain and help you manage your weight.

Stress:

Stress is closely connected to weight gain. When you are stressed, your body releases the stress hormone cortisol. Studies indicate that cortisol promotes the storage of body fat in the abdominal area. Also, stress makes you likely to consume more food as a coping mechanism. You need to learn how to manage stress properly by performing relaxation techniques and regularly taking time off from work.

Menopause:

During menopause, certain hormone levels decrease in the body of the woman. This can cause changes in body composition and its ability to burn calories. This can also increase the menopausal woman's appetite which leads to weight gain. The metabolism also slows down during this stage of a woman's life making weight loss difficult.

Television:

There are many studies showing that watching several hours of television a day can make you more prone to gaining weight. This is especially the case when you eat in front of the television. Eating while watching TV has been found to significantly increase the amount of food consumed. It would be much better to eat in your dining area so that you will be able to completely concentrate on your food. This will help you feel full faster and eat less.

Lifestyle Factors:

One of the main causes of weight gain is a person's lifestyle. Alcoholic beverages contain a high amount of calories so even moderate indulgence can lead to weight gain. An inactive lifestyle also makes you more prone to gaining weight.

Weight Loss

Weight loss refers to the reduction in the total mass of the body due to a loss of body fat, fluid or lean mass. It is caused due to malnourishment or due to an underlying medical condition. In some cases, weight loss is generated through a conscious effort by adhering to a work-out regime or a diet to improve health and fitness or to change the appearance of the body. In cases where weight loss is unexplained, or does not correspond to a reduction in calorific intake or exercise, an underlying medical condition may be the most obvious reason.

Weight loss is desirable for over-weight or obese individuals as it delays diabetes, reduces pain and increases mobility in people with osteoarthritis of the knee, reduces hypertension, besides others. The most recommended weight loss technique that is the least intrusive, involves increased physical activity and adjustments to eating patterns. Reducing processed food that is high in sugar, saturated fats and salt can aid the weight loss process. Intake of supplements and drugs for reducing appetite or stomach volume and blocking fat absorption may also be considered alternative weight loss strategies. In case of severe obesity, surgical interventions may be performed, such as gastric bypass and gastric banding. These options are ideally not considered healthy techniques as they come with a set of associated risks and complications. There exists a substantial market for weight loss products from self-help books to body belts and cremes to supplements. It is wise to weigh the pros and cons of the multitude of choices available and instead make smart choices in terms of basic lifestyle changes.

Causes of Weight Loss

Cancer

In the vast majority of cases of cancer, other symptoms will develop before any weight loss. There are many symptoms that can occur, depending on the type and site of the cancer. However, occasionally, weight loss is the first symptom noticed. The weight loss is partly due to the increased activity of cancer cells in the body that require nutrition. (Weight loss in more advanced cancer is due to various combined factors.)

Type 2 Diabetes

Type 2 diabetes occurs mainly in people aged over 40 although it can occur at younger ages. The four common symptoms are being thirsty a lot of the time, passing large amounts of urine, tiredness and weight loss. Some people pass off the first three symptoms to do with other things, or 'getting older'. So, weight loss is sometimes the first thing reported to a doctor. The weight loss is partly due to the sugar (glucose) that is passed out with the urine.

Depression

Depression has a number of symptoms. However, some people do not recognise that they have depression. They may feel low and not right but cannot say why. They may even think of it as just normal for them. Many people with depression can hide their true feelings from friends and family. Weight loss may develop due to not eating much. It is sometimes friends or family who may actually notice that a person has lost weight and it then turns out to be due to depression.

Alcohol Abuse/Alcohol Dependence

Some people who drink a lot of alcohol do not look after themselves very well. Their diet may not be very good and they may lose weight. However, they may be in denial about an alcohol problem. It may be friends or family who actually notice that the person has lost weight. Indeed, this is a way that a hidden alcohol problem in some people comes to light. Family and friends may show concern about weight loss and not be aware that the person has an alcohol problem.

Hyperthyroidism

Hyperthyroidism means that you make too much of a hormone called thyroxine. The extra thyroxine causes many of your body's functions to speed up. There are lots of possible symptoms such as:

- Being restless.
- Being nervous or anxious.
- Being more emotional.
- Being irritable.
- Sleeping poorly.
- Having the sensation of a 'thumping heart' (palpitations).

- Shaking (tremor).
- Sweating more.
- Loose and/or frequent stools (diarrhoea).
- Being 'always on the go'.

Another typical symptom is losing weight despite an increased appetite. This may be a first symptom. But, again, some of the other symptoms that may occur such as being restless, nervous, emotional or irritable may just be put down to a stressful time of life or to your personality. In the early stages of hyperthyroidism some people actually feel well and full of energy and don't realise they have a problem but lose weight.

Persistent (Chronic) Infection or Inflammation

It would be unusual not to have other symptoms with a chronic infection. But, occasionally, the first symptom that is noticed with infections such as tuberculosis or HIV is weight loss. Hookworm infection of the gut is another example where weight loss may be the first indication of disease. Hookworm is a very common problem worldwide (but rare in the UK). Likewise, there are various conditions that cause persistent inflammation of a part or parts of the body. Again, other symptoms would be usual. But, sometimes an inflammatory condition such as polymyalgia rheumatica may just make you feel unwell and lose weight prior to other symptoms developing.

Malabsorption Syndromes

There are various diseases that can affect the way food is absorbed and taken into the body from the gut. These would normally cause symptoms such as diarrhoea. However, weight loss may be the first symptom noticed. Examples include coeliac disease, Crohn's disease and ulcerative colitis.

Dementia

People in the early stages of dementia may appear to get by reasonably well but, in fact, they are not able to look after themselves very well. They may have a poor diet but appear happy in themselves. Again, it is sometimes friends or family who may first notice that a person is not right and has lost weight and it then turns out to be the early stages of dementia.

Eating Disorders

In conditions such as anorexia, a person usually knows they are tightly controlling their diet and exercise and are actively trying to lose weight. However, this may be hidden from friends and family and may not be divulged even to the doctor.

Side-effects from Medication

Sometimes medication may cause side-effects resulting in weight loss. For example, some pills may cause a loss of appetite, or a dry mouth. Some cause heartburn or give a mild tummy discomfort. Others may affect the sense of taste or smell, or make people feel sick. Any of these side-effects could affect eating habits and result in a loss of weight.

Caloric Restriction

Caloric restriction is an experimental tool that utilizes "undernutrition without malnutrition." In other words, caloric restriction means lowering typical calorie consumption by 30 to 40 percent, while maintaining all the necessary nutrients and vitamins to support life. Until recently, researchers found this to be the only reliable way to increase longevity in mammals. Two new studies, however, have shown that a diet containing very low levels of an amino acid called methionine can also extend lifespan in mice and rats.

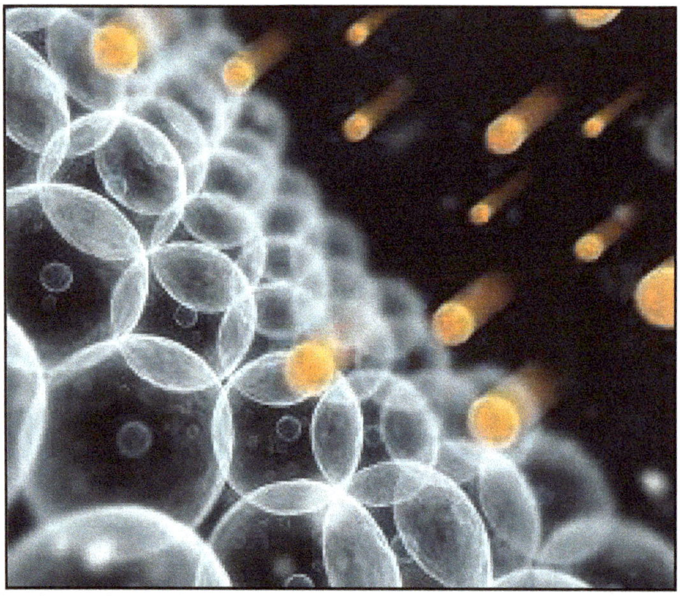

Caloric restriction has been observed to retard and even reverse oxidative damage in aging animals. Oxidative damage is caused when free radicals and peroxides bombard cells.

The Importance of Caloric Restriction

Caloric restriction has been shown to increase both the average and the maximal lifespan in paramecia (creatures made of a single cell), worms, spiders, insects, and rodents. Non-human primates are now being tested, but the complete outcome of these tests will not be known for several decades because monkeys have relatively long lifespans compared to other animals. Preliminary results suggest that calorie-restricted monkeys are healthier and tend to live longer than their freely fed counterparts. For example, one new study shows that the immune systems of aged rhesus monkeys on a calorie restricted diet resembles, in several ways, the immune systems of younger animals.

Although caloric restriction diets are so difficult to maintain that they are unlikely to be a practical approach to delayed aging for people, studying the mechanisms of calorie restriction is still very important. Caloric restriction seems to prevent or delay many age-associated diseases and conditions, such as heart disease, dementia, and cancer. If scientists can figure out how it works, they might be able to develop drugs that mimic its effects without requiring people to drastically reduce their calorie intake and risk potentially dangerous side effects.

Caloric restriction may or may not extend the total number of years a human can expect to live, but of equal or greater importance, perhaps, is the possibility of adding to the number of years we can expect to remain healthy. Reducing or delaying age-related diseases until the very end of life would represent an enormous improvement in quality of life for many, if not most, older adults.

The Role of Caloric Restriction in Aging

Caloric restriction seems to slow down some of the destructive processes that take place in cells and tissues as they age. Scientists don't yet know exactly how or why it works, but they have developed several theories.

First, caloric restriction seems to reduce damage from chemicalmetabolic processes, particularly oxidative and glycation damage,thought to be leading causes of cell aging and death.

On a larger scale, caloric restriction slows the effects of aging on the nervous system, the reproductive organs, and the production of hormones in some animals. It has also been shown to delay the onset of certain age-related cancers. However, whether or not CR enhances or decreases immune function has not been resolved.

Health Effects

In humans, the long-term health effects of moderate caloric restriction with sufficient nutrients are unknown.

Risks of Malnutrition

The term "calorie restriction" as used in gerontology refers to dietary regimens that reduce calorie intake without incurring malnutrition. If a restricted diet is not designed to include essential nutrients, malnutrition may result in serious deleterious effects, as shown in the Minnesota Starvation Experiment. This study was conducted during World War II on a group of lean men, who restricted their calorie intake by 45% for 6 months and composed roughly 77% of their diet with carbohydrates. As expected, this malnutrition resulted in many positive metabolic adaptations (e.g. decreased body fat, blood pressure, improved lipid profile, low serum T3 concentration, and decreased resting heart rate and whole-body resting energy expenditure), but also caused a wide range of negative effects, such as anemia, edema, muscle wasting, weakness, neurological deficits, dizziness, irritability, lethargy, and depression.

Musculoskeletal Losses

Short-term studies in humans report a loss of muscle mass and strength and reduced bone mineral density. However, whether or not the reduction in bone mineral density actually harms bone health is unclear. In a study in premenopausal women, bone mineral density after weight loss was higher when normalized for body weight; reduced bone mineral density is also observed in humans undergoing long-term calorie restriction with adequate nutrition, but no fractures have been reported and the reduction in bone mineral density was not associated with deleterious changes in bone microarchitecture.

Lower-than-normal Body Mass Index, High Mortality

Caloric restriction diets typically lead to reduced body weight, yet reduced weight can come from other causes and is not in itself necessarily healthy. In some studies, low body weight has been associated with increased mortality, particularly in late middle-aged or elderly subjects. Low body weight in the elderly can be caused by pathological conditions associated with aging and predisposing to higher mortality (such as cancer, chronic obstructive pulmonary disorder, or depression) or of the cachexia (wasting syndrome) and sarcopenia (loss of muscle mass, structure, and function). One of the more famous of such studies linked a body mass index lower than 18 in women with increased mortality from noncancer, non–cardiovascular disease causes. The authors attempted to adjust for confounding factors (cigarette smoking, failure to exclude pre-existing disease); others argued that the adjustments were inadequate.

> "epidemiologists from the ACS (American Cancer Society), American Heart Association, Harvard School of Public Health, and other organizations raised specific methodologic questions about the recent Centers for Disease Control and Prevention study and presented analyses of other data sets. The main concern is that it did not adequately account for weight loss from serious illnesses such as cancer and heart disease and failed to account adequately for the effect of smoking on weight As a result, the Flegal study underestimated the risks from obesity and overestimated the risks of leanness."

Such epidemiological studies of body weight are not about caloric restriction as used in anti-aging studies; they are not about caloric intake to begin with, as body weight is influenced by many factors other than energy intake, Moreover, "the quality of the diets consumed by the low-body mass index individuals are difficult to assess, and may lack nutrients important to longevity." Typical low-calorie diets rarely provide the high nutrient intakes that are a necessary feature of an anti-aging calorie restriction diet. As well, "The lower-weight individuals in the studies are not a caloric restriction because their caloric intake reflects their individual ad libitum set-points and not a reduction from that set-point."

Triggering Binge Eating

In those who have a binge-eating disorder, calorie restriction can precipitate an episode of binge eating, but it does not seem to pose any such risk otherwise.

Young or Pregnant

Long-term caloric restriction at a level sufficient for slowing the aging process is generally not recommended in children, adolescents, and young adults (under the age of approximately 21), because this type of diet may interfere with natural physical growth, as has been observed in laboratory animals. In addition, mental development and physical changes to the brain take place in late adolescence and early adulthood that could be negatively affected by severe caloric restriction. Pregnant women and women trying to become pregnant are advised not to practice calorie restriction, because low BMI may result in ovulatory dysfunction (infertility), and underweight mothers are more prone to preterm delivery.

Miscellaneous Concerns

It has also been noted that people losing weight on such diets risk developing cold sensitivity, menstrual irregularities, infertility, and hormonal changes.

Mechanisms

Even though there has been research on caloric restriction for over 70 years, the mechanism by which caloric restriction works is still not well understood. Some explanations include reduced core body temperature, reduced cellular divisions, lower metabolic rates, reduced production of free radicals, reduced DNA damage and hormesis.

Temperature

Caloric restriction lowers the core body temperature, a phenomenon believed to be an adaptive response to reduce energy expenditure when nutrients availability is limited.

Lowering the temperature may prolong the lifespan of cold blooded animals. Mice, which are warm blooded, have been engineered to have a reduced core body temperature which increased the lifespan independently of calorie restriction.

Hormesis

Some research has pointed toward hormesis as an explanation for the benefits of caloric restriction, representing beneficial actions linked to a low-intensity biological stressor such as reduced calorie intake. As a potential role for caloric restriction, the diet imposes a low-intensity biological stress on the organism, eliciting a defensive response that may help protect it against the disorders of aging. In other words, caloric restriction places the organism in a defensive state so that it can survive adversity, resulting in improved health and longer life. This switch to a defensive state may be controlled by longevity genes.

Mitochondrial Hormesis

Mitochondrial hormesis was a purely hypothetical concept until late 2007, when work on a small worm named Caenorhabditis elegans suggested that the restriction of glucose metabolism extends life span primarily by increasing oxidative stress to stimulate the organism into having an ultimately increased resistance to further oxidative stress. This is probably the first experimental evidence for hormesis being the reason for extended life span following caloric restriction.

Although aging can be conceptualized as the accumulation of damage, the more recent determination that free radicals participate in intracellular signaling has made the categorical equation of their effects with "damage" more problematic than was commonly appreciated in the past. It was previously proposed on a hypothetical basis that free radicals may induce an endogenous response culminating in more effective adaptations that protect against exogenous radicals (and possibly other toxic compounds). Sublethal mitochondrial stress with an attendant augmentation of reactive oxygen species may precipitate many of the beneficial alterations in cellular physiology produced by caloric restriction.

Evolution

It has been recently argued that during years of famine, it may be evolutionarily desirable for an organism to avoid reproduction and to up-regulate protective and repair enzyme mechanisms to ensure that it is fit for reproduction in future years. This argument seems to be supported by recent work studying hormones. Prolonged severe CR lowers total serum and free testosterone while increasing sex hormone binding globulin concentrations in humans; these effects are independent of adiposity.

Lowering of the concentration of insulin and substances related to insulin, such as insulin-like growth factor 1 and growth hormone, has been shown to up-regulate autophagy, the repair mechanism of the cell. A related hypothesis suggests that caloric restriction works by decreasing insulin levels and thereby up-regulating autophagy, but caloric restriction affects many other health indicators, and it is still undecided whether insulin is the main concern. Calorie restriction has been shown to increase DHEA in primates, but it has not been shown to increase DHEA in post-pubescent primates. The extent to which these findings apply to humans is still under investigation.

Chromatin and PHA-4

Evidence suggests that the biological effects of caloric restriction are closely related to chromatin function. One study determined that the gene PHA-4 is responsible for the longevity behind calorie restriction in roundworms, "with similar results expected in humans".

Reduced DNA Damage

Calorie restriction reduces production of reactive oxygen species.

Sohal et al. observed that caloric restriction decreased 8-OHdG damages in the DNA of mice heart, skeletal muscle, brain, liver and kidney. The levels of 8-OHdG in the DNA of these organs in 15 month old mice were reduced to an average of 81% of that in the DNA of mice fed an unrestricted diet. Kaneko et al. observed that, in rats, dietary restriction retarded the onset of age-related increases in 8-OHdG in nuclear DNA of brain, heart, liver and kidney. The level of 8-OHdG in these organs of the calorie restricted rats at 30 months averaged 65% of the level in rats fed an unrestricted diet.

In rodents, calorie restriction slows aging, decreases ROS production and reduces the accumulation of oxidative DNA damage in multiple organs. These results link reduced oxidative DNA damage to slower aging. The consistent observation that calorie restriction reduces oxidative DNA damage lends support to the possibility that oxidative DNA damage is associated with aging.

Sirtuin-mediated Mechanism

Preliminary research indicates that sirtuins are activated by fasting and serve as "energy sensors" during metabolism. Sirtuins, specifically Sir2 (found in yeast) have been implicated in the aging of yeast, and are a class of highly conserved, NAD^+-dependent histone deacetylase enzymes. Sir2 homologs have been identified in a wide range of organisms from bacteria to humans. Yeast has 3 SIR genes (SIR2, SIR3, and SIR4) that are responsible for silencing mating type loci, telomeres, and rDNA. Although all three genes are required for the silencing of mating type loci and telomeres, only SIR2 has been implicated in the silencing of rDNA. In addition, SIR2 related genes also regulate formation of some specialized survival forms, such as spores in yeast and daher larvae in *C. elegans*. A study done by Kaeberlein et al. (1999) in yeast found that deletions of Sir2 decreased lifespan, and additional copies increased lifespan.

In many calorie restriction studies, it is believed that Sir2 mediates the longevity effects from calorie restriction for several reasons. First, it was found that in yeast without SIR2, calorie restriction did not impart longevity in yeast; second, in Sir2 mutants an abundance of extra-chromosomal ribosomal DNA circles (that typically limit lifespan) has been observed, and that mitigation of these circles restore regular life span, but still are resistant to calorie restriction-mediated longevity; third, that caloric restriction increases the activity of Sir2 *in vivo*. Although Sir2 has been implicated in calorie restriction-mediated longevity, the method by which Sir2 is regulated under caloric restriction is still debated.

Two hypotheses of Sir2/caloric restriction-mediated longevity is the NADH mechanism and the NAD salvage pathway mechanism. In the NADH hypothesis, it is believed that caloric restriction causes an increase in respiration, which in turn causes a reduction in the levels of NADH. This decrease in the concentration of NADH would up regulate SIR2, since NADH functions as a competitive inhibitor of SIR2. In addition, it has been shown that overexpression of NADH hydrogenase increased longevity and knocking out the electron transport chain blocked caloric restriction-mediated longevity. The NAD salvage pathway mechanism relies on a study by Anderson et al., in which they showed that caloric restriction causes an up regulation of PNC1 (an enzyme responsible for synthesizing NAD from nicotinamide and ADP-ribose) decreases the levels of nicotinamide, which in turn upregulates SIR2 and thus increases lifespan. Although these models are not mutually exclusive, no experiment has been conducted linking the two.

Caloric Restriction Mimetics

Work on the mechanisms of caloric restriction has given hope to the synthesizing of future drugs to increase the human lifespan by simulating the effects of calorie restriction. In particular, the large number of genes and pathways reported to regulate the actions of caloric restriction in model organisms represent attractive targets for developing drugs that mimic the benefits of CR without its side effects.

Sir2, or "silent information regulator 2", is a sirtuin, discovered in baker's yeast cells, that is hypothesized to suppress DNA instability. In mammals, Sir2 is known as SIRT1. One proponent of the view that the gene Sir2 may underlie the effect of calorie restriction in mammals by protecting cells from dying under stress. It is suggested that a low-calorie diet that requires less Nicotinamide adenine dinucleotide to metabolize may allow SIRT1 to be more active in its life-extending processes, possibly by a mechanism of SIRT1 releasing fat from storage cells.

Sirtuins

Attempts are being made to develop drugs that act as CR mimetics, and much of that work has focused on a class of proteins called sirtuins. Resveratrol has been reported to activate SIRT1 and extend the lifespan of yeast, nematode worms, fruit flies, vertebrate fish, and mice consuming a high-caloric diet. However, resveratrol does not extend life span in normal mice and the effect of resveratrol on lifespan in nematodes and fruit flies has been disputed.

There are studies that indicate that resveratrol may not function through SIRT1 but may work through other targets. A clinical trial of the resveratrol formulation SRT501 was suspended.

Caloric Restriction Mimetic

Although the beneficial effects of caloric restriction on lifespan and health have been clearly demonstrated, it is difficult to implement such restrictions in our lives. To overcome these difficulties, gerontologists and biologists are attempting to develop drugs to mimic the beneficial effects of caloric restriction without the need for diet limitations. Such medicines are known as caloric restriction mimetics (CRM).

Resveratrol

Resveratrol is a polyphenol compound isolated from the skins of red grapes. Resveratrol is currently the most thoroughly studied CRM. As a CRM, resveratrol was first identified by Sinclair through screening of small molecular libraries for compounds that activate Sirtuin and extend lifespan in a yeast model. In that study, they demonstrated that resveratrol can mimic the benefits associated with caloric restriction, and that caloric restriction did not further extend the lifespan of yeast grown in resveratrol supplemented medium. Resveratrol was subsequently shown to extend longevity in worms, flies, fish, and obese mice. However, a recent study showed that resveratrol had no effect on the longevity of mice fed a normal diet. Although the longevity extension effect of resveratrol is not yet certain, it is accepted that resveratrol can improve health and prevent age-related diseases. Further investigations and clarifications are required to verify whether resveratrol is a true CRM.

Rapamycin

Rapamycin, an antibiotic, immune-suppressor drug, is another proposed CRM that has shown a longevity benefit. After studies showing the extension of replicative lifespan of yeast via inhibition of the TOR signaling in response to rapamycin treatment, it was reported that rapamycin extends the median and maximum lifespan of 20-month-old mice accompanied with a decrease in TOR activity. Since then, many studies have been conducted to ascertain the function of rapamycin as a CRM. However, it is important to note that there is evidence showing adverse side-effects of rapamycin such as an increase in the incidence of diabetes.

Metformine

Metformin is another CRM of interest to gerontologists. Metformin is a biguanide used as a drug for treatment of type-2 diabetes that increases insulin sensitivity and activates AMPK. Metformin received a great deal of attention after it was identified in a screening assay of drugs showing similar transcriptional profiles to that of caloric restriction in mice. Moreover, metformin was shown to have a caloric restriction-related longevity benefit mediated by the activation of AMPK in *C. elegans*. Metformin also has a beneficial effect on other aspects of the aging process such as a decrease in age-related disease incidence. However, the longevity benefit of metformin was not observed in a *Drosophila* model in a recent study, or in the non-disease rodent model. The appearance of evidence showing that metformin is ineffective on longevity in some species has led to uncertainty as to whether metformin is a true CRM.

Meal Replacement

The term "meal replacement" generally refers to a calorie-controlled, prepackaged product in the form of a bar or beverage (ready to drink or powder), that replaces a regular meal.

Meal-replacement products usually provide 200 to 250 calories per serving, are fortified with more than 20 vitamins and minerals at "good" or "excellent source" levels and often bear nutrient content claims, such as percent fat free and reduced sugar.

Some meal replacement products use the term "meal" in the statement of identity, while others use the term only in romance copy and advertising to recommend uses: "occasional meal replacement," "meal supplement" or "snack."

Initially, meal replacement products were consumed mainly by elderly or ill adults, frequently with nutritional deficiencies. In recent years, however, the marketing of meal replacements has increasingly targeted healthy adults. Such products are presented as a convenient source of balanced nutrition or for specific purposes including weight loss, maintenance and gain.

Proponents tout the nutritional advantages of meal replacements over "empty" calorie alternatives and believe the calorie-controlled portions can be beneficial for weight loss and maintenance.

Critics discourage reliance on meal replacements, other than on an occasional basis, because such usage may decrease the servings of so-called "real food" like fruits and vegetables. Studies by the American Institute for Cancer Research and similar groups show fruits and vegetables are a greater source of antioxidant protection than supplements alone, as well as providing the additional health benefits of phytochemicals.

Another concern raised by critics is that consumers using meal replacements as a main source of nutrition, unless supervised by a medical professional, may not consume sufficient calories or nutrients, depending on the formulation.

Regulation of Meal Replacements

Meal replacement products can be regulated as conventional/functional foods. Those represented as weight-loss products sometimes include warnings, particularly if the product is specifically labeled as a "meal." The packaging may also suggest a weight control plan, with meal replacements substituting for one meal per day (for weight maintenance) or two meals per day (for weight loss), in addition to snacks.

Regulations also mandate information and statements that must be given on the labels of foods for special dietary use. The label of a product represented to be for special dietary use with respect to reducing or maintaining weight must bear a conspicuous statement of the basis upon which the food claims to be of special dietary usefulness. Foods for special dietary use are subject to nutrition labeling and health claim requirements, like conventional/functional foods.

Another regulatory category covering meal replacements is medical foods. These are foods specially formulated to be consumed or administered enterally under active, ongoing medical supervision, and intended for the dietary management of a specific disease or condition for which distinctive nutritional requirements are established by medical evaluation. Medical foods are not intended for use by the general public, and are primarily available through hospitals, clinics and other medical facilities. Medical foods are exempt from nutrition labeling and health claim requirements.

Meal Replacement Diets Advantages

1. Easy to follow – you don't need to plan menus, shop for exotic ingredients or do much in the way of weighing and measuring to follow a meal replacement diet; simply whip up a shake and drink instead of eating a regular meal. This makes them ideal for people who are always on the go or who don't really know what they should eat to lose weight.
2. Time-efficient – how many times have you said that you don't have time to prepare and cook and healthy, fat-fighting meal? With meal replacement shakes, your meal is ready in seconds; great for busy people.

3. Convenient – most shakes can be prepared in advance and carried with you to work or to school so there is no reason to fall off the "diet wagon" because you don't have your diet meal with you. Many shakes are also available pre-mixed or are made from dry ingredients and easily mixed with water when required making them very transportable.
4. Balanced – containing all the nutrients you need, meal replacement shakes are often healthier than exclusion diets such as Atkins or other diets where entire food groups are banned.
5. Fast fat loss – one of the most noteworthy aspects of this type of diet is they produce fast results. Granted, some of the rapid initial fat loss will be water but fat loss is rapid too.
6. Adaptable – you can speed up or slow down fat loss to suit your needs by adjusting the number of shakes you have per day. For very rapid fat loss, you might consume nothing but shakes for a few days and limit yourself to just a couple of solid food meals per week. This may be necessary if you are getting in shape for a competition of some kind or simply want to look your best for a big event e.g. a wedding. Alternatively, if you are in less of a rush to lose weight or have less to lose, you might have two shakes and two solid food meals per day.

Meal Replacement Diets Disadvantages

1. Can be socially exclusive – your family are sitting down to their regular meal and you have your shake to drink; this may mean you don't want to join them at meal times. If you usually eat with your family or friends this can result in feelings of social exclusion at meal times.
2. Can be boring – food is one of life's great pleasures and while a shake can be tasty and enjoyable, it's not the same as a "real" meal. Shake-based diets can get very old very quickly unless you can find ways to make your shakes more exciting and interesting. For that reason, some meal replacement diets also include things like meal replacement bars and even soups.
3. May lack fiber – fiber is an important substance for digestive health that is found in grains, fruits and vegetables. While most meal replacement shakes contain some fiber, it might not be enough to keep your digestive system healthy. Generally, you need between 25 and 35 grams of fiber per day and if your chosen shake does not provide this, you may need to consider taking a fiber supplement. This is easily remedied, however, by adding fruits, vegetables or even oatmeal to meal replacement shakes or you can add something like psyllium husks which are a good source of calorie-free fiber too.
4. Do not promote healthy eating habits – weight gain is inevitably caused by eating too much of the wrong foods and this is often down to simply not knowing

what foods to eat and when. Meal replacement diets fix the symptom of weight gain but do not really address the long term causes. Once you have finished your meal replacement diet and go back to your old eating regimen, you will probably regain some or even all of the weight you have lost unless you modify your eating habits.

5. Not suitable for long term use – meal replacement diets are not really suitable for long term use. You'll soon get bored of drinking so many similar-tasting shakes and as nutritionally balanced as the shakes usually are, they are not as complete as real food. Your body needs real food.
6. Expense – some shakes are very expensive and may even work out more costly than eating a regular, healthy diet. This can mean that some people start a meal replacement diet but are then unable to continue because of the cost. This is especially true of pre-mixed products. Thankfully, and just for you, we have come up with a way to make meal replacement diets more affordable.

References

- Woodhouse R (2008). "Obesity in art: a brief overview". Frontiers of Hormone Research. Frontiers of Hormone Research. 36: 271–86. doi:10.1159/000115370. ISBN 978-3-8055-8429-6. PMID 18230908
- Sweeting HN (October 2007). "Measurement and definitions of obesity in childhood and adolescence: a field guide for the uninitiated". Nutrition Journal. 6 (1): 32. doi:10.1186/1475-2891-6-32. PMC 2164947. PMID 17963490
- "Antibiotics: repeated treatments before the age of two could be a factor in obesity". Prescrire International. 2018. Retrieved 2 July2018
- Kushner R (2007). Treatment of the Obese Patient (Contemporary Endocrinology). Totowa, NJ: Humana Press. p. 158. ISBN 1-59745-400-1. Retrieved April 5, 2009
- Salmon J, Timperio A (2007). "Prevalence, trends and environmental influences on child and youth physical activity". Medicine and Sport Science (Review). Medicine and Sport Science. 50: 183–99. doi:10.1159/000101391. ISBN 978-3-318-01396-2. PMID 17387258
- Weinstock, Matthew (June 21, 2013). "The Facts About Obesity". H&HN. American Hospital Association. Retrieved June 24, 2013

5

Doping in Sports

Doping or the use of performance enhancing drugs is a widespread phenomenon in sports. Performance enhancing drugs are substances used illicitly to improve athletic performance. This chapter sheds light on such practices and its side effects as well as the various measures, such as doping tests, taken to prevent it.

A performance enhancing drug is any drug that has the potential to change the human body and its functions in such a way to improve athletic performance. Ideally, the PED would increase the body function in such a way as to give the taker of the drug a marked advantage over their non-doping competition.

While the rewards of winning may be great, PED use actually comes with significant health risks, including death in some cases. PEDs can be classified into groups based on what type of chemical they are and the effect the drug has on the human body.

Following are the common types of performance enhancing drugs:

Anabolic Steroids

Some athletes take a form of steroids — known as anabolic-androgen steroids or just anabolic steroids — to increase their muscle mass and strength. The main anabolic steroid hormone produced by your body is testosterone.

Testosterone has two main effects on your body:

- Anabolic effects promote muscle building.
- Androgenic effects are responsible for male traits, such as facial hair and a deeper voice.

Some athletes take straight testosterone to boost their performance. Frequently, the anabolic steroids that athletes use are synthetic modifications of testosterone.

These hormones have approved medical uses, though improving athletic performance is not one of them. They can be taken as pills, injections or topical treatments.

Why are these drugs so appealing to athletes? Besides making muscles bigger, anabolic steroids may help athletes recover from a hard workout more quickly by reducing the muscle damage that occurs during the session. This enables athletes to work out harder and more frequently without overtraining. In addition, some athletes may like the aggressive feelings they get when they take the drugs.

Designer Steroids

A particularly dangerous class of anabolic steroids are the so-called designer drugs — synthetic steroids that have been illicitly created to be undetectable by current drug tests. They are made specifically for athletes and have no approved medical use. Because of this, they haven't been tested or approved by the Food and Drug Administration (FDA) and represent a particular health threat to athletes.

Risks of Designer Steroids

Many athletes take anabolic steroids at doses that are much higher than those prescribed for medical reasons, and most of what is known about the drugs' effects on athletes comes from observing users.

It is impossible for researchers to design studies that would accurately test the effects of large doses of steroids on athletes, because giving participants such high doses would be unethical. This means that the effects of taking anabolic steroids at very high doses haven't been well-studied.

Anabolic steroids come with serious physical side effects as well. Men may develop:

- Prominent breasts,
- Baldness,
- Shrunken testicles,
- Infertility,
- Impotence,
- Prostate gland enlargement.

Women may develop:

- A deeper voice,
- An enlarged clitoris,
- Increased body hair,
- Baldness,
- Infrequent or absent periods.

Both men and women might experience:

- Severe acne.
- Increased risk of tendinitis and tendon rupture.
- Liver abnormalities and tumors.
- Increased low-density lipoprotein (LDL) cholesterol (the "bad" cholesterol).
- Decreased high-density lipoprotein (HDL) cholesterol (the "good" cholesterol).
- High blood pressure (hypertension).
- Heart and circulatory problems.
- Aggressive behaviors, rage or violence.
- Psychiatric disorders, such as depression.
- Drug dependence.
- Infections or diseases such as HIV or hepatitis if you're injecting the drugs.
- Inhibited growth and development, and risk of future health problems in teenagers.

Taking anabolic-androgenic steroids to enhance athletic performance, besides being prohibited by most sports organizations, is illegal. In the past 20 years, more effective law enforcement in the United States has pushed much of the illegal steroid industry into the black market.

This poses additional health risks because the drugs are either made in other countries and smuggled in or made in clandestine labs in the United States. Either way, they aren't subject to government safety standards and could be impure or mislabeled.

Androstenedione

Androstenedione (andro) is a hormone produced by the adrenal glands, ovaries and testes. It's a hormone that's normally converted to testosterone and estradiol in both men and women. Andro is available legally only in prescription form and is a controlled substance.

Manufacturers and bodybuilding magazines tout its ability to allow athletes to train harder and recover more quickly. However, its use as a performance-enhancing drug is illegal in the United States.

Scientific studies that refute these claims show that supplemental androstenedione doesn't increase testosterone and that your muscles don't get stronger with andro use.

Risks of Androstenedione

Side effects of andro in men include:

- Acne.
- Diminished sperm production.
- Shrinking of the testicles.
- Enlargement of the breasts.

In women, side effects include:

- Acne.
- Masculinization, such as deepening of the voice and male-pattern baldness.

In both men and women, andro can decrease HDL cholesterol (the "good" cholesterol), which puts you at greater risk of heart attack and stroke.

Human Growth Hormone

Human growth hormone, also known as gonadotropin, is a hormone that has an anabolic effect. Athletes take it to improve muscle mass and performance. However, it hasn't been shown conclusively to improve either strength or endurance. It is available only by prescription and is administered by injection.

Risks of Human Growth Hormone

Adverse effects related to human growth hormone range in severity and may include:

- Joint pain.
- Muscle weakness.
- Fluid retention.
- Vision problems.
- Carpal tunnel syndrome.
- Impaired glucose regulation.
- Enlarged heart (cardiomegaly).
- High cholesterol (hyperlipidemia).
- Diabetes.
- High blood pressure (hypertension).

Erythropoietin

Erythropoietin is a type of hormone used to treat anemia in people with severe kidney disease. It increases production of red blood cells and hemoglobin, resulting in improved movement of oxygen to the muscles. Epoetin, a synthetic form of erythropoietin, is commonly used by endurance athletes.

Risks of Erythropoietin

Erythropoietin use among competitive cyclists was common in the 1990s and allegedly contributed to at least 18 deaths. Inappropriate use of erythropoietin may increase the risk of thrombotic events, such as stroke, heart attack and pulmonary embolism.

Diuretics

Diuretics are drugs that change your body's natural balance of fluids and salts (electrolytes) and can lead to dehydration. This loss of water can decrease an athlete's weight, helping him or her to compete in a lighter weight class, which many athletes prefer. Diuretics may also help athletes pass drug tests by diluting their urine and are sometimes referred to as a "masking" agent.

Risks of Diuretics

Diuretics taken at any dose, even medically recommended doses, predispose athletes to adverse effects such as:

- Dehydration,
- Muscle cramps,
- Dizziness,
- Potassium deficiency,
- Rash,
- Gout,
- Drop in blood pressure,
- Loss of coordination and balance,
- Death.

Creatine

Many athletes take nutritional supplements instead of or in addition to performance-enhancing drugs. Supplements are available over-the-counter as powders or pills. The most popular supplement among athletes is probably creatine monohydrate.

Creatine is a naturally occurring compound produced by your body that helps your muscles release energy. Scientific research indicates that creatine may have some athletic benefit by producing small gains in short-term bursts of power.

Creatine appears to help muscles make more adenosine triphosphate (ATP), which stores and transports energy in cells, and is used for quick bursts of activity, such as weightlifting or sprinting. There's no evidence, however, that creatine enhances performance in aerobic or endurance sports.

Your liver produces about 0.07 ounces (2 grams) of creatine each day. You also get creatine from the meat in your diet.

Creatine is stored in your muscles, and levels are relatively easily maintained. Because your kidneys remove excess creatine, the value of supplements to someone who already has adequate muscle creatine content is questionable.

Risks of Creatine

Supplements are considered food and not drugs by the FDA. This means supplement manufacturers are not required to conform to the same standards as drug manufacturers do. In some cases, supplements have been found to be contaminated with other substances, which may inadvertently lead to a positive test for performance-enhancing drugs.

Possible side effects of creatine that can decrease athletic performance include:

- Stomach cramps,
- Muscle cramps,
- Weight gain.

Weight gain is sought after by athletes who want to increase their size. But with prolonged creatine use, weight gain is more likely the result of water retention than an increase in muscle mass. Water is drawn into your muscle tissue, away from other parts of your body. This puts you at risk of dehydration.

High-dose creatine use may potentially damage your:

- Kidneys,
- Liver.

It appears safe for adults to use creatine at the doses recommended by manufacturers. But there are no studies investigating the long-term benefits and risks of creatine supplementation.

Stimulants

Some athletes use stimulants to stimulate the central nervous system and increase heart rate and blood pressure.

Stimulants can:

- Improve endurance.
- Reduce fatigue.
- Suppress appetite.
- Increase alertness and aggressiveness.

Common stimulants include caffeine and amphetamines. Cold remedies often contain the stimulants ephedrine or pseudoephedrine hydrochloride.

Energy drinks, which are popular among many athletes, often contain high doses of caffeine and other stimulants. The street drugs cocaine and methamphetamine also are stimulants.

Risks of Stimulants

Although stimulants can boost physical performance and promote aggressiveness on the field, they have side effects that can impair athletic performance.

- Nervousness and irritability, which make it hard to concentrate on the game.
- Insomnia, which can prevent an athlete from getting needed sleep.
- Dehydration.
- Heatstroke.
- Addiction or tolerance, meaning that athletes need greater amounts to achieve the desired effect, so they'll take doses that are much higher than the intended medical dose.

Other side effects include:

- Heart palpitations.
- Heart rhythm abnormalities.
- Weight loss.
- Tremors.
- Mild high blood pressure (hypertension).
- Hallucinations.

- Stroke.
- Heart attack and other circulatory problems.

Endurance Sports

The use of performance-enhancing drugs in sport has become an increasing problem across a wide range of sports. It is defined as any substance or drug that, when taken, gives an athlete an unfair advantage relative to a "clean" athlete. The banning of these drugs promotes a level playing field and equality among athletes. The use of 'the suit' in swimming, which gives athletes an advantage in the way of hydrodynamics, has been banned from international competition due to the unfair advantage it delivered. The drugs taken by athletes differ widely based on the performance needs of the sport.

Erythropoietin (EPO) is largely taken by endurance athletes who seek a higher level of red blood cells, which leads to more oxygenated blood, and a higher VO2 max. An athlete's VO2 max is highly correlated with success within endurance sports such as swimming, long-distance running, cycling, rowing, and cross-country skiing. EPO has recently become prevalent amongst endurance athletes due to its potentcy and low degree of detectability when compared to other methods of doping such as blood transfusion. While EPO is believed to have been widely used by athletes in the 1990s, there was not a way to directly test for the drug until 2002 as there was no specific screening process to test athletes . Athletes at the Olympic Games are tested for EPO through blood and urine tests. Stringent guidelines and regulations can lessen the danger of doping that has existed within some endurance sports.

Non-endurance Sports

In sports where physical strength is favored, athletes have used anabolic steroids, known for their ability to increase physical strength and muscle mass. The drug mimics the effect of testosterone and dihydrotestosterone in the body. They were developed after Eastern Bloc countries demonstrated success in weightlifting during the 1940s. At the time they were using testosterone, which carried with it negative effects, anabolic steroids were developed as a solution. The drug has been used across a wide range of sports from football and basketball to weightlifting and track and field. While not as life-threatening as the drugs used in endurance sports, anabolic steroids have negative side effects, including:

Side Effects in Men

- acne.
- impaired liver function.
- impotency.

- breast formation (gynecomastia).
- increase in estrogen.
- erectile dysfunction.
- increased sex drive.
- male pattern baldness.
- risk of heart failure.

Side Effects in Women

Side effects in women include:

- hair loss.
- male pattern baldness.
- hypertrophy of the clitoris.
- increased sex drive.
- irregularities of the menstrual cycle.
- development of masculine facial traits.
- increased coarseness of the skin.
- premature closure of the epiphysis.
- deepening of the voice.

In countries where the use of these drugs is controlled, there is often a black market trade of smuggled or counterfeit drugs. The quality of these drugs may be poor and can cause health risks. In countries where anabolic steroids are strictly regulated, some have called for a regulatory relief. Steroids are available over-the-counter in some countries such as Thailand and Mexico.

Reaction from Sports Organizations

Many sports organizations have banned the use of performance-enhancing drugs and have very strict rules and penalties for people who are caught using them. The International Amateur Athletic Federation, now the International Association of Athletics Federations, were the first international governing body of sport to take the situation seriously. In 1928 they banned participants from doping, but with little in the way of testing available they had to rely on the word of the athlete that they were clean. It was not until 1966 that FIFA and Union Cycliste Internationale (cycling) joined the IAAF in the fight against drugs, followed by the International Olympic Committee the following year. Progression in pharmacology has always outstripped the ability of sports federations to implement rigorous testing procedures but since the creation of the World Anti-Doping Agency in 1999, it has become more effective to catch athletes who use drugs. The first tests for athletes were at the 1966 European Championships and two years later the IOC implemented their first drug tests at both the Summer and Winter Olympics. Anabolic steroids became prevalent during the 1970s and after a method of detection was found they were added to the IOC's prohibited substances list in 1975.

Over the years, different sporting bodies have evolved differently in the struggle against doping. Some, such as athletics and cycling, are becoming increasingly vigilant against doping. However, there has been criticism that sports such as football (soccer) and baseball are doing nothing about the issue, and letting athletes implicated in doping away unpunished.

Some commentators maintain that, as outright prevention of doping is an impossibility, all doping should be legalised. However, most disagree with this, pointing out the claimed harmful long-term effects of many doping agents. Opponents claim that with doping legal, all competitive athletes would be compelled to use drugs, and the net effect would be a level playing field but with widespread health consequences. Considering that anti-doping is largely ineffective due to both testing limitations and lack of enforcement, this is not markedly different from the situation already in existence.

Another point of view is that doping could be legalized to some extent using a drug whitelist and medical counseling, such that medical safety is ensured, with all usage published. Under such a system, it is likely that athletes would attempt to cheat by exceeding official limits to try to gain an advantage; this could be considered conjecture as drug amounts do not always correlate linearly with performance gains.

Blood Doping

Blood doping is an illicit method of improving athletic performance by artificially boosting the blood's ability to bring more oxygen to muscles.

In many cases, blood doping increases the amount of hemoglobin in the bloodstream. Hemoglobin is an oxygen-carrying protein in the blood. So increasing hemoglobin allows higher amounts of oxygen to reach and fuel an athlete's muscles. This can improve stamina and performance, particularly in long-distance events, such as running and cycling.

Blood doping is banned by the International Olympic Committee and other sports organizations.

Blood doping is defined as the use of illicit products (e.g. erythropoietin (EPO), darbepoetin-alfa, hypoxia-inducible factor (HIF) stabilizers) and methods (e.g. increase aerobic capacity by maximizing the uptake of O_2) in order to enhance the O_2 transport of the body to the muscles.

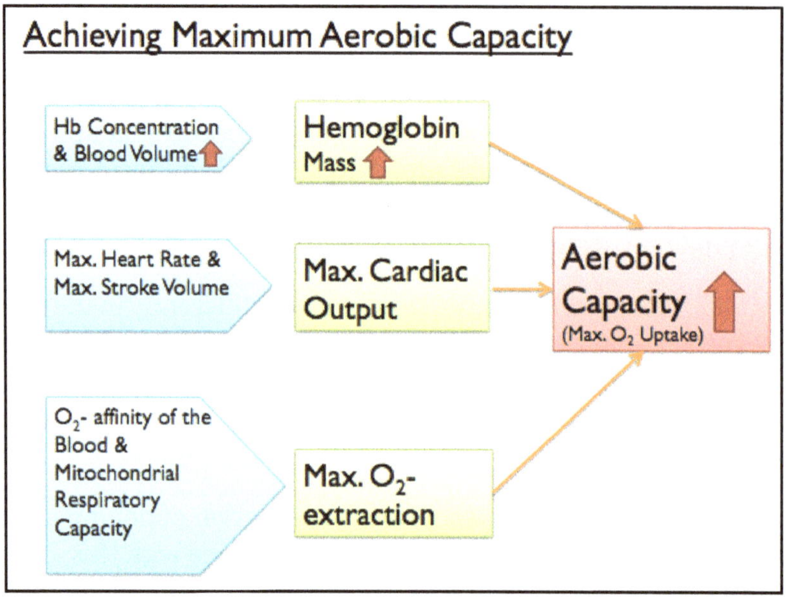

Achieving Maximum Aerobic Capacity.

The body undergoes aerobic respiration in order to provide sufficient delivery of O_2 to the exercising skeletal muscles and the main determining factors are shown in figure above. The rate of maximum O_2 uptake (O_2max) depends on cardiac output, O_2 extraction and hemoglobin mass. The cardiac output of an athlete is difficult to manipulate during competitions and the distribution of cardiac output is at the maximum rate (i.e. 80%) during competitions. In addition, the O_2 extraction is approximately 90% at maximal exercise. Therefore, the only method to enhance the physical performance left is to increase the O_2 content in the artery by enhancing the hemoglobin mass. In other words, hemoglobin concentration and blood volume contribute to hemoglobin mass.

Methods

Drug Treatments

Many forms of blood doping stem from the misuse of pharmaceuticals. These drug treatments have been created for clinical use to increase the oxygen delivery when the human body is not able to do so naturally.

Erythropoietin

Erythropoietin (EPO) is a glycoprotein hormone produced by the interstitial fibroblasts in the kidney that signal for erythropoiesis in bone marrow. The increased activity of a Hemocytoblast (RBC stem cell) allows the blood to have a greater carrying capacity for oxygen. EPO was first developed to counteract the effects of chemotherapy and radiation therapy for cancer patients. EPO also stimulates increased wound healing.

Because of its physiological side effects, particularly increased hematocrit, EPO has become a drug with abuse potential by professional and amateur cyclists.

Hypoxia-inducible Factor (HIF) Stabilizer

Hypoxia-inducible factor stabilizer (HIF stabilizer) is a pharmaceutical used to treat chronic kidney disease. Like most transcription factors, the HIF transcription factor is responsible for the expression of a protein. The HIF stabilizer activates the activity of EPO due to anemia induced hypoxia, metabolic stress, and vasculogenesis—the creation of new blood vessels. HIF stabilizers as used by cyclists in combination with cobalt chloride/desferrioxamine stimulate and de-regulate the natural production of erythropoietin hormone. At physiologically low PaO_2 around 40 mmHg, EPO is released from the kidneys to increase hemoglobin transportation. The combination of drugs consistently releases EPO due to increased transcription at the cellular level. The effect wears off when the HIF stabilizers, cobalt chloride/desferrioxamine is excreted and/or decayed by the body.

Myo-inositol Trispyrophosphate (ITPP)

Myo-inositol trispyrophosphate (ITPP), also known as compound number OXY111A, is an allosteric effector of hemoglobin which causes a rightward shift in the oxygen–hemoglobin dissociation curve, increasing the amount of oxygen released from red blood cells into surrounding tissue during each passage through the cardiovascular system. ITPP has been a subject of anti-doping research in both humans and racehorses.

Blood Transfusion

Blood transfusions can be traditionally classified as autologous, where the blood donor and transfusion recipient are the same, or as allogeneic/homologous, where the blood is transfused into someone other than the donor. Blood transfusion begins by the withdrawal of 1 to 4 units of blood (1 unit = 450 ml of blood) several weeks before competition. The blood is centrifuged, the plasma components are immediately reinfused, and the corpuscular elements, principally red blood cells (RBCs), are stored refrigerated at 4 °C or frozen at −80 °C. As blood stored by refrigeration displays a steady decline in the number of RBCs, a substantial percentage, up to 40%, of the stored RBCs may not be viable. The freezing process, conversely, limits the aging of the cells, allowing the storage of the blood for up to 10 years with a 10% to 15% loss of RBCs. Stored RBCs are then reinfused, usually 1 to 7 days before a high-endurance event. As a significant amount of iron is removed by each autologous transfusion, an adequate time for recovery of not less than 3 days from the last donation, and appropriate iron supplements, are usually required for patients undergoing autologous donations. Nearly 50% of autologous donations are not used by the donor and are discarded, as current standards do not allow transfusion of these units to another patient for safety reasons.

Blood Substitutes

Biochemical and biotechnological development has allowed novel approaches to this issue, in the form of engineered O_2 carriers, widely known as “blood substitutes.” The blood substitutes currently available are chiefly polymerized haemoglobin solutions or haemoglobin-based oxygen carriers (HBOCs) and perfluorocarbons (PFCs).

Hemoglobin-based Oxygen Carriers (HBOCs)

Hemoglobin-based oxygen carriers are intra/ inter-molecularly engineered human or animal hemoglobins, only optimized for oxygen delivery and longer intravascular circulation. The presence of 2,3-diphosphoglycerate within erythrocytes maintains the normal affinity of hemoglobin for oxygen. HBOCs do not contain erythrocytes and lose this interaction, thus, unmodified human HBOC solutions have a very high oxygen affinity which compromises their function. Chemical methods developed to overcome this problem have resulted in carriers that effectively release oxygen at the physiological pO_2 of peripheral tissues.

A common feature of all HBOCs is their resistance to dissociate when dissolved in media, which contrasts hemoglobin of natural dissociation under non-physiological conditions. HBOCs may hypothetically supply greater benefits to athletes than those provided by the equivalent hemoglobin in traditional RBC infusion. Recent developments have shown that HBOCs are not only simple RBC substitutes, but highly effective O_2 donors in terms of tissue oxygenation. Additional effects include increases in blood serum iron, ferritin, and Epo; up to 20% increased diffusion of oxygen and improved exercise capacity; increased CO_2 production; and lower lactic acid generation in anaerobic activity. HBOCs been shown in trials to be extreemly dangerous in humans. Because Haemoglobin-based oxygen carriers increase both the risk of death and risk of myocardial infarction clinical trials were ended. They are not commercially available in the US or Europe and there is no approved use for them.

Perfluorocarbons (PFCs)

PFCs, also known as fluorocarbons, are inert, water-insoluble, synthetic compounds, consisting primarily of carbon and fluorine atoms bonded together in strong C–F bonds. PFCs are substantially clear and colorless liquid emulsions that are heterogeneous in molecular weight, surface area, electronic charge, and viscosity; their high content of electron-dense fluorine atoms results in little intramolecular interaction and low surface tension, making such substances excellent solvents for gases, especially oxygen and carbon dioxide. Some of these molecules can dissolve 100 times more oxygen than plasma. PFCs are naturally hydrophobic and need to be emulsified to be injected intravenously. Since PFCs dissolve rather than bind oxygen, their capacity to serve as a blood substitute is determined principally by the pO_2 gradients in the lung and at the target tissue. Therefore, their oxygen transport properties differ substantially from those of whole blood and, especially, from those of RBCs. At a conventional ambient pO_2 of 135 mmHg, the oxygen content of 900 ml/l perfluorocarbon is less than 50 ml/l, whereas an optimal oxygen content of 160 ml/l, which is still lower than that of whole blood in normal conditions, can be achieved only by a pO_2 greater than 500 mmHg. In practice, at a conventional alveolar pO_2 of 135 mmHg, PFCs will not be able to provide sufficient oxygenation to peripheral tissues.

Due to their small size, PFCs are able to permeate circulation where erythrocytes may not flow. In tiny capillaries, PFCs produce the greatest benefit, as they increase local oxygen delivery much more efficiently than would be expected from the increase in oxygen content in larger arteries. In addition, as gases are in the dissolved state within PFCs, it pO_2 promotes efficient oxygen delivery to peripheral tissues. Since the mid-1980s, improvements in both oxygen capacity and emulsion properties of PFCs have led to the development of second-generation PFCbased oxygen carriers; two PFC products are currently being tested in phase III clinical trials.

Cobalt Chloride Administration

Transition metal complexes are widely known to play important roles in erythropoiesis; as such, inorganic supplementation is proving to be an emerging technique in blood doping. Particularly of note is the cobalt complex, cobalamin (Vitamin B_{12}) commonly used as a dietary supplement. Cobalamin is an important complex used in the manufacture of red blood cells and thus was of interest for potential use in blood doping. Experimental evidence, however, has shown that cobalamin has no effect on erythropoiesis in the absence of a red blood cell/oxygen deficiency. These results seem to confirm much of what is already known about the functioning of cobalamin. The signaling pathway that induces erythropoietin secretion and subsequently red blood cell manufacture using cobalamin is O_2 dependent. Erythropoietin is only secreted in the kidneys when there is an O_2 deficiency, as such, RBC manufacture is independent of the amount of cobalamin administered when there is no O_2 deficiency. Accordingly, cobalamin is of little to no value in blood doping.

More potent for use in blood doping is Co^{2+} (administered as Cobalt(II) chloride, $CoCl_2$). Cobalt chloride has been known to be useful in treating anemic patients. Recent experimental evidence has proved the efficacy of cobalt chloride in blood doping. Studies into the action of this species have shown that Co^{2+} induces hypoxia like responses, the most relevant response being erythropoiesis. Co^{2+} induces this response by binding to the N-terminus (loop helix loop domain) of the Hypoxia inducing transcription factors HIF-1α and HIF-2α, and thus stabilizes these protein complexes. Under normal O_2 conditions, HIFs are destabilized as proline and asparagine residues are hydroxylated by HIF-α hydroxylases, these unstable HIFs are subsequently degraded following a ubiquitin-proteosome pathway, as such, they cannot then bind and activate transcription of genes encoding Erythropoietin (EPO). With Co^{2+} stabilization, degradation is prevented and genes encoding EPO can then be activated. The mechanism for this Co^{2+} N terminus stabilization is not yet fully understood. In addition to N-terminus binding, it has also been hypothesized that replacement of Fe^{2+} by Co^{2+} in the hydroxylase active site could be a contributing factor to the stabilizing action of Co^{2+}. It is understood however, is that Co^{2+} binding permits Ubiquitin binding but prevents proteosomal degradation.

Notable Blood Doping Cases

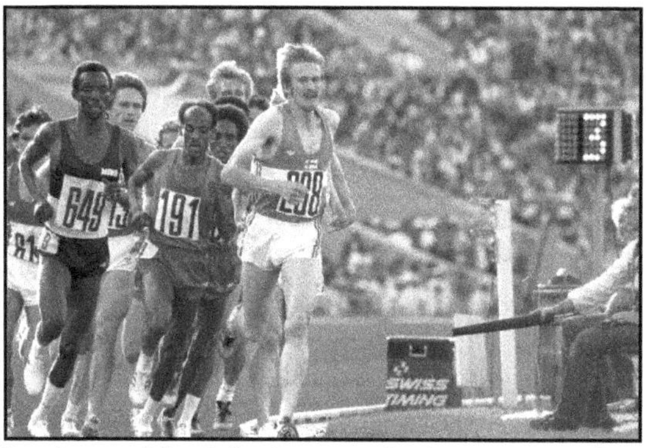

The subject of the first known blood doping case, in the Summer Olympics 5,000 m race.

Blood doping started in the late 1960s but was not outlawed until 1986. While it was still legal, it was commonly used by middle and long-distance runners. The first known case of blood doping occurred at the 1980 Summer Olympics in Moscow as Kaarlo Maaninka was transfused with two pints of blood before winning medals in the 5 and 10 kilometer track races, though this was not against the rules at the time. Cyclist Joop Zoetemelk admitted to receiving blood transfusions during the 1976 Tour de France, where he finished second, although he claimed that these were intended to treat his anaemia rather than enhance his performance. The American cyclist Pat McDonough admitted to blood doping at the 1984 Summer Olympics in Los Angeles. Following the 1984 Summer games it was revealed that one-third of the U.S. cycling team had received blood transfusions before the games, where they won nine medals, their first medal success since the 1912 Summer Olympics. In the same year cyclist Francesco Moser used blood transfusions to prepare for his successful attempt to break the hour record. "Blood doping" was banned by the IOC in 1985, though no test existed for it at the time.

The Swedish cyclist Niklas Axelsson tested positive for EPO in 2000.

The American cyclist Tyler Hamilton failed a fluorescent-activated cell sorting test for detecting homologous blood transfusions during the 2004 Olympics. He was allowed to keep his gold medal because the processing of his sample precluded conducting a second, confirmatory test. He appealed a second positive test for homologous transfusion from the 2004 Vuelta a España to the International Court of Arbitration for Sport but his appeal was denied. Hamilton's lawyers proposed Hamilton may be a genetic chimera or have had a 'vanishing twin' to explain the presence of red blood cells from more than one person. While theoretically possible, these explanations were ruled to be of "negligible probability".

The Spanish-based Operación Puerto case in 2006 involved allegations of doping and blood doping of hundreds of athletes from Spain, Germany, Italy, Colombia, Australia, Luxembourg, The Netherlands and The USA.

Tour de France rider Alexander Vinokourov, of the Astana Team, tested positive for two different blood cell populations and thus for homologous transfusion, according to various news reports on July 24, 2007. Vinokourov was tested after his victory in the 13th stage time trial of the Tour on July 21, 2007. A doping test is not considered to be positive until a second sample is tested to confirm the first. Vinokourov's B sample has now tested positive, and he faces a possible suspension of 2 years and a fine equal to one year's salary. He also tested positive after stage 15.

Vinokourov's teammate Andrej Kashechkin also tested positive for homologous blood doping on August 1, 2007, just a few days after the conclusion of the 2007 Tour de France (a race that had been dominated by doping scandals). His team withdrew after the revelation that Vinokourov had doped.

According to Russian investigators, 19-year-old New York Rangers prospect and Russian hockey player Alexei Cherepanov was engaged in blood doping for several months before he died on October 13, 2008, after collapsing on the bench during a game in Russia. He also had myocarditis.

The German speed skater and five-fold Olympic gold medalist Claudia Pechstein was banned for two years in 2009 for alleged blood doping, based on irregular levels of reticulocytes in her blood and the assumption that these levels were always highest during competitions. Her mean reticulocyte count over the ten years from 2000 to 2009 was 2.1% during top events like Olympic Games and during world championships. At world cup races the mean reticulocyte was 1.9% and during training phases 2.0%. The Court of Arbitration for Sport confirmed the ban in November 2009 in stating: "once the possibility of a blood disease has been safely excluded". In September 2010, the Swiss Federal Supreme Court rejected the athlete's appeal, stating that Pechstein's inherited blood anomaly had been known before ("die vererbte Blutanomalie bekannt gewesen sei").

On May 20, 2011 Tyler Hamilton turned in his 2004 Olympic Gold Medal to the U.S. Anti-Doping Agency after admitting to doping in a *60 Minutes* interview.

On August 23, 2012 Lance Armstrong was stripped of his seven Tour de France titles and banned for life by cycling's governing body following a report from the U.S. Anti-Doping Agency that accused him of leading a doping program during his cycling career. He later admitted to using banned substances including blood doping with transfusions and EPO in an interview with Oprah Winfrey on January 17, 2013.

In June 2014, UFC fighter Chael Sonnen tested positive for EPO. One month later, another UFC fighter, Ali Bagautinov also tested positive for EPO.

In December 2017, Russia was banned from the 2018 Winter Games in Pyeongchang, South Korea due to systematic doping among Russian Olympians.

Adverse Effects

The simple act of increasing the number of red blood cells in blood may be associated with hyperviscosity syndrome which is characterized by increased blood viscosity and decreased cardiac output and blood flow velocity which results in the reduction of peripheral oxygen delivery. For instance, an overdose of EPO can thicken blood into a highly viscous and artery-clogging sludge. This increases the chances of heart attack, stroke, phlebitis, and pulmonary embolism, which has been seen in cases where there is too much blood reintroduced into the blood stream. Because blood doping increases the volume of red blood cells, it effectively introduces a condition called polycythemia, a blood disorder that has known adverse outcomes such as heart attacks or strokes.

Blood contamination during preparation or storage is another issue. Contamination was seen in 1 in every 500,000 transfusions of red blood cells in 2002. Blood contamination can lead to septicemia or an infection that affects the whole body.

Certain medications used to increase red blood cells can reduce liver function and lead to liver failure, pituitary problems, and increases in cholesterol levels.

What will happen if a person takes more than one drug?

As complex interactions can occur among various types of drugs, the side effects of taking a combination of drugs are likely to be much more severe and serious and thus increase the risk of a harmful or fatal outcome.

Are drugs addictive? Will they cause permanent health damage?

Yes, drugs can create both physical and psychological dependence. When the drug is discontinued, withdrawal symptoms may occur as a result of this dependence. Prolonged use of large dosages of performance enhancing substances may also cause permanent and irreversible side effects.

Doping Testing

Doping testing is an activity that is strictly specified in the International Standard for Testing and Investigations. Urine, blood or both are collected as test samples. Doping testing takes place both at competitions and outside of them.

Doping Test Types

There are two types of doping tests: in-competition tests and out-of-competition tests. An athlete can be summoned to testing at any time and anywhere, either in their home country or abroad. The athlete is invited in person.

In-competition Tests

In-competition tests refer to doping tests performed in connection with a competition event. Unless otherwise specified in the rules of the international or another relevant antidoping organisation, this refers to a period starting 12 hours prior to the competition and ending at the end of the competition and the related collection of samples.

All known doping substances and methods and any manipulation of the sample are tested from samples collected in connection with competitions.

The athletes are drawn or ordered to undergo testing based on ranking, for example, or chosen for it as specified in the competition rules of the sport. The athletes can also be ordered to take the test by name in the in-competition tests.

In some sports, a record result (Finnish record, European record, world record) cannot be officially approved until the athlete in question has produced a negative sample. After breaking a record, the athlete must attend the doping control in a manner provided by the rules of the sport. The athlete can acquire further information from his or her sports federation.

Out-of-competition Tests

Targeted doping tests are also carried out outside of competitions. Out-of-competition samples are tested for non-approved substances, anabolic agents, peptide hormones, growth factors and similar substances, ß2-agonists, hormone and metabolism modulators, diuretics and other masking agents as well as all prohibited methods.

International sports federations may have rules of their own regarding the substances to be tested. It is the athletes responsibility to be aware of the relevant rules.

Athletes are chosen for out-of-competition tests in a targeted manner or by drawing the athletes to be tested during the training of a certain group or athletes on a camp. In targeted tests, FINADA or another antidoping organisation that has ordered the test has named the athlete in advance for the test.

Targeted tests are mainly carried out for testing pool and national team athletes. FINADA can, however, target any athlete bound by the antidoping code for testing, both in-competition and out-of-competition.

Out-of-competition tests also include follow-up tests made to clarify the results of previous tests and tests carried out during a period of ineligibility due to antidoping rule violations.

Types

Urine Drug Screen

Urine analysis is primarily used because of its low cost. Urine drug testing is one of the most common testing methods used. The enzyme-multiplied immune test is the most frequently used urinalysis. Complaints have been made about the relatively high rates of false positives using this test.

Urine drug tests screen the urine for the presence of a parent drug or its metabolites. The level of drug or its metabolites is not predictive of when the drug was taken or how much the patient used. Rather, it is simply a confirmatory report indicating the presence of the parent drug or its metabolites.

Urine drug testing is an immunoassay based on the principle of competitive binding. Drugs which may be present in the urine specimen compete against their respective drug conjugate for binding sites on their specific antibody. During testing, a urine specimen migrates upward by capillary action. A drug, if present in the urine specimen below its cut-off concentration, will not saturate the binding sites of its specific antibody. The antibody will then react with the drug-protein conjugate and a visible colored line will show up in the test line region of the specific drug strip.

When an employer requests a drug test from an employee, or a physician requests a drug test from a patient, the employee or patient is typically instructed to go to a collection site or their home. The urine sample goes through a specified 'chain of custody' to ensure that it is not tampered with or invalidated through lab or employee error. The patient or employee's urine is collected at a remote location in a specially designed secure cup, sealed with tamper-resistant tape, and sent to a testing laboratory to be screened for drugs (typically the Substance Abuse and Mental Health Services Administration 5 panel). The first step at the testing site is to split the urine into two aliquots. One aliquot is first screened for drugs using an analyzer that performs immunoassay as the initial screen. To ensure the specimen integrity and detecting possible adulterant, some other parameters such as, urine creatinine, pH, and specific gravity are tested along in this initial test. If the urine screen is positive then another aliquot of the sample is used to confirm the findings by gas chromatography—mass spectrometry (GC-MS) or liquid chromatography - mass spectrometry methodology. If requested by the physician or employer, certain drugs are screened for individually; these are generally drugs part of a chemical class that are, for one of many reasons, considered more abuse-prone or of concern. For instance, oxycodone and diamorphine may be tested, both sedative analgesics. If such a test is not requested specifically, the more general test (in the preceding case, the test for opiates) will detect the drugs, but the employer or physician will not have the benefit of the identity of the drug.

Employment-related test results are relayed to a medical review office (MRO) where a medical physician reviews the results. If the result of the screen is negative, the MRO informs the employer that the employee has no detectable drug in the urine, typically within 24 hours. However, if the test result of the immunoassay and GC-MS are non-negative and show a concentration level of parent drug or metabolite above the established limit, the MRO contacts the employee to determine if there is any legitimate reason—such as a medical treatment or prescription.

On-site instant drug testing is a more cost-efficient method of effectively detecting drug abuse amongst employees, as well as in rehabilitation programs to monitor patient progress. These instant tests can be used for both urine and saliva testing. Although the accuracy of such tests varies with the manufacturer, some kits boast extremely high rates of accuracy, correlating closely with laboratory test results.

Breath Test

Breath test is a widespread method for quickly determining alcohol intoxication. A breath test measures the alcohol concentration in the body by a deep-lung breath. There are different instruments used for measuring the alcohol content of an individual though their breath. Breathalyzer is a widely known instrument which was developed in 1954 and contained chemicals unlike other breath-testing instruments. More modernly used instruments are the infrared light-absorption devices and fuel cell detectors, these two testers are microprocessor controlled meaning the operator only has to press the start button.

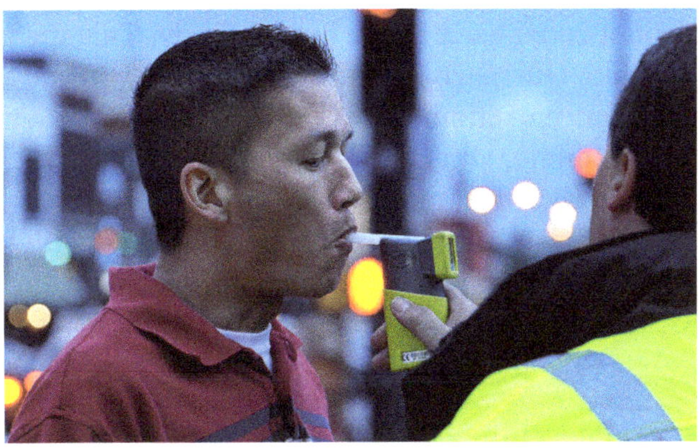

Breath test being used on a volunteer.

To get accurate readings on a breath-testing device the individual must blow for approximately 6 seconds and need to contain roughly 1.1 to 1.5 liters of breath. For a breath-test to result accurately and truly an operator must take steps such as avoiding measuring "mouth alcohol" which is a result from regurgitation, belching, or recent intake of an alcoholic beverage. To avoid measuring "mouth alcohol" the operator must not allow the individual that's taking the test to consume any materials for at least fifteen minutes before the breath test. When pulled over for a driving violation if an individual in the United States refuses to take a breath test that individual's driver's license can be suspend for a 6 to 12 months time period.

Hair Testing

Hair analysis to detect drugs of abuse has been used by court systems in the United States, United Kingdom, Canada, and other countries worldwide. In the United States, hair testing has been accepted in court cases as forensic evidence following the Frye Rule, the Federal Rules of Evidence, and the Daubert Rule. As such, hair testing results are legally and scientifically recognized as admissible evidence.

Although some lower courts may have accepted hair test evidence, there is no controlling judicial ruling in either the federal or any state system declaring any type of hair test as reliable.

Hair testing is now recognized in both the UK and US judicial systems. There are guidelines for hair testing that have been published by the Society of Hair Testing (a private company in France) that specify the markers to be tested for and the cutoff concentrations that need to be tested. Drugs of abuse that can be detected include Cannabis, Cocaine, Amphetamines and drugs new to the UK such as Mephedrone.

Alcohol

In contrast to other drugs consumed, alcohol is deposited directly in the hair. For this reason the investigation procedure looks for direct products of ethanol metabolism. The main part of alcohol is oxidized in the human body. This means it is released as water and carbon dioxide. One part of the alcohol reacts with fatty acids to produce esters. The sum of the concentrations of four of these fatty acid ethyl esters (FAEEs: ethyl myristate, ethyl palmitate, ethyl oleate and ethyl stearate) are used as indicators of the alcohol consumption. The amounts found in hair are measured in nanograms (one nanogram equals only one billionth of a gram), however with the benefit of modern technology, it is possible to detect such small amounts. In the detection of ethyl glucuronide, or EtG, testing can detect amounts in picograms (one picogram equals 0.001 nanograms).

However, there is one major difference between most drugs and alcohol metabolites in the way in which they enter into the hair: on the one hand like other drugs FAEEs enter into the hair via the keratinocytes, the cells responsible for hair growth. These cells form the hair in the root and then grow through the skin surface taking any substances with them. On the other hand, the sebaceous glands produce FAEEs in the scalp and these migrate together with the sebum along the hair shaft. So these glands lubricate not only the part of the hair that is just growing at 0.3 mm per day on the skin surface, but also the more mature hair growth, providing it with a protective layer of fat.

FAEEs (nanogram = one billionth of a gram) appear in hair in almost one order of magnitude lower than (the relevant order of magnitude of) EtG (picogram = one trillionth of a gram). It has been technically possible to measure FAEEs since 1993, and the first study reporting the detection of EtG in hair was done by Sachs in 1993.

In practice, most hair which is sent for analysis has been cosmetically treated in some way (bleached, permed etc.). It has been proven that FAEEs are not significantly affected by such treatments. FAEE concentrations in hair from other body sites can be interpreted in a similar fashion as scalp hair.

Presumptive Substance Testing

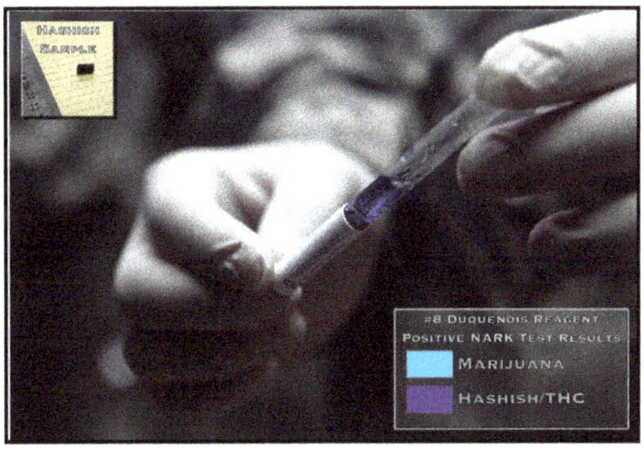

Duquenois reagent

Presumptive substance tests identify a suspicious substance, material or surface where traces of drugs are thought to be, instead of testing individuals through biological methods such as urine or hair testing. The test involves mixing the suspicious material with a chemical in order to trigger a color change to indicate if a drug is present. Most are now available over-the-counter, and do not require a lab to read results.

Benefits to this method include that the person who is suspected of drug use does not need to be confronted or aware of testing. Only a very small amount of material is needed to obtain results, and can be used to test powder, pills, capsules, crystals, or organic material. There is also the ability to detect illicit material when mixed with other non-illicit materials. The tests are used for general screening purposes, offering a generic result for the presence of a wide range of drugs, including Heroin, Cocaine, Methamphetamine, Amphetamine, Ecstasy/MDMA, Methadone, Ketamine, PCP, PMA, DMT, MDPV, and may detect rapidly evolving synthetic designer drugs. Separate tests for Marijuana/Hashish are also available.

There are five primary color-tests reagents used for general screening purposes. The Marquis reagent turns into a variety of colors when in the presence of different substances. Dille-Koppanyi reagent uses two chemical solutions which turns a violet-blue color in the presence of barbiturates. Duquenois-Levine reagent is a series of chemical solutions that turn to the color of purple when the vegetation of marijuana is added. Van Urk reagent turns blue-purple when in the presence of LSD. Scott Test's chemical solution shows up as a faint blue for cocaine base.

Saliva Drug Screen / Oral Fluid-based Drug Screen

Saliva / oral fluid-based drug tests can generally detect use during the previous few days. Is better at detecting very recent use of a substance. THC may only be detectable for 2–24 hours in most cases. On site drug tests are allowed per the Department of Labor.

Detection in saliva tests begins almost immediately upon use of the following substances, and lasts for approximately the following times:

- Alcohol: 6-12 h.
- Marijuana: 1-24h.

A disadvantage of saliva based drug testing is that it is not approved by FDA or SAMHSA for use with DOT / Federal Mandated Drug Testing. Oral fluid is not considered a bio-hazard unless there is visible blood; however, it should be treated with care.

Sweat Drug Screen

Sweat patches are attached to the skin to collect sweat over a long period of time (up to 14 days). These are used by child protective services, parole departments, and other government institutions concerned with drug use over long periods, when urine testing is not practical. There are also surface drug tests that test for the metabolite of parent drug groups in the residue of drugs left in sweat.

Blood

Drug-testing a blood sample measures whether or not a drug or a metabolite is in the body at a particular time. These types of tests are considered to be the most accurate way of telling if a person is intoxicated. Blood drug tests are not used very often because they need specialized equipment and medically trained administrators.

Depending on how much marijuana was consumed, it can usually be detected in blood tests within six hours of consumption. After six hours has passed, the concentration of marijuana in the blood decreases significantly. It generally disappears completely within 30 days.

Anabolic Steroids

Anabolic steroids are used to enhance performance in sports and as they are prohibited in most high-level competitions drug testing is used extensively in order to enforce this prohibition. This is particularly so in individual (rather than team) sports such as athletics and cycling.

Random Drug Testing

Can occur at any time, usually when the investigator has reason to believe that a substance is possibly being abused by the subject by behavior or immediately after an employee-related incident occurs during work hours. Testing protocol typically conforms to the national medical standard, candidates are given up to 120 minutes to reasonably produce a urine sample from the time of commencement (in some instances this time frame may be extended at the examiners discretion).

Diagnostic Screening

In the case of life-threatening symptoms, unconsciousness, or bizarre behavior in an emergency situation, screening for common drugs and toxins may help find the cause, called a *toxicology test* or *tox screen* to denote the broader area of possible substances beyond just self-administered drugs. These tests can also be done post-mortem during an autopsy in cases where a death was not expected. The test is usually done within 96 hours (4 days) after the desire for the test is realized. Both a urine sample and a blood sample may be tested. A blood sample is routinely used to detect ethanol/methanol and ASA/paracetamol intoxication. Various panels are used for screening urine samples for common substances, e.g. *triage 8* that detects amphetamines, benzodiazepines, cocaine, methadone, opiates, cannabis, barbiturates and tricyclic antidepressants. Results are given in 10–15 min.

Similar screenings may be used to evaluate the possible use of date rape drugs. This is usually done on a urine sample.

Methodologies

Before testing samples, the tamper-evident seal is checked for integrity. If it appears to have been tampered with or damaged, the laboratory rejects the sample and does not test it.

Next, the sample must be made testable. Urine and oral fluid can be used "as is" for some tests, but other tests require the drugs to be extracted from urine. Strands of hair, patches, and blood must be prepared before testing. Hair is washed in order to eliminate second-hand sources of drugs on the surface of the hair, then the keratin is broken down using enzymes. Blood plasma may need to be separated by centrifuge from blood cells prior to testing. Sweat patches are opened and the sweat collection component is removed and soaked in a solvent to dissolve any drugs present.

Laboratory-based drug testing is done in two steps. The first step is the screening test, which is an immunoassay based test applied to all samples. The second step, known as the confirmation test, is usually undertaken by a laboratory using highly specific chromatographic techniques and only applied to samples that test positive during the screening test. Screening tests are usually done by immunoassay (EMIT, ELISA, and RIA are the most common). A "dipstick" drug testing method which could provide screening test capabilities to field investigators has been developed at the University of Illinois.

After a suspected positive sample is detected during screening, the sample is tested using a confirmation test. Samples that are negative on the screening test are discarded and reported as negative. The confirmation test in most laboratories (and all SAMHSA certified labs) is performed using mass spectrometry, and is precise but expensive. False positive samples from the screening test will almost always be negative on the confirmation test. Samples testing positive during both screening and confirmation tests are reported as positive to the entity that ordered the test. Most laboratories save positive samples for some period of months or years in the event of a disputed result or lawsuit. For workplace drug testing, a positive result is generally not confirmed without a review by a Medical Review Officer who will normally interview the subject of the drug test.

Urine Drug Testing

Urine drug test kits are available as on-site tests, or laboratory analysis. Urinalysis is the most common test type and used by federally mandated drug testing programs and is considered the Gold Standard of drug testing. Urine based tests have been upheld in most courts for more than 30 years. However, urinalysis conducted by the Department of Defense has been challenged for reliability of testing the metabolite of cocaine. There are two associated metabolites of cocaine, benzoylecgonine (BZ) and ecgonine methyl ester (EME), the first (BZ) is created by the presence of cocaine in an aqeous solution with a pH greater than 7.0, while the second (EME) results from the actual human metabolic process. The presence of EME confirms actual ingestion of cocaine by a human being, while the presence of BZ is indicative only. BZ without EME is evidence of sample contamination, however, the US Department of Defense has chosen not to test for EME in its urinalysis program.

A number of different analyses (defined as the unknown substance being tested for) are available on Urine Drug Screens.

Spray Drug Testing

Spray (sweat) drug test kits are non-invasive. It is a simple process to collect the required specimen, no bathroom is needed, no laboratory is required for analysis, and the tests themselves are difficult to manipulate and relatively tamper-resistant. The detection window is long and can detect recent drug use within several hours.

There are also some disadvantages to spray or sweat testing. There is not much variety in these drug tests, only a limited number of drugs can be detected, prices tend to be higher, and inconclusive results can be produced by variations in sweat production rates in donors. They also have a relatively long specimen collection period and are more vulnerable to contamination than other common forms of testing.

Hair Drug Testing

Hair drug testing is a method that can detect drug use over a much longer period of time, and is often used for highly safety-critical positions where there is zero tolerance of illegal drug use. Standard hair follicle screen covers a period of 30 to 90 days. The growth of hair is usually at the rate of 0.5 inches per month. The hair sample is cut close to the scalp and 80 to 120 strands of hair are needed for the test. In the absence of hair on the head, body hair can be used as an acceptable substitute. This includes facial hair, the underarms, arms, and legs or even pubic hair. Because body hair grows at a different rate than head hair, the timeframe changes, with scientists estimating that drug use can be detected in body hair for up to 12 months. Currently, most entities that use hair testing have prescribed consequences for individuals removing hair to avoid a hair drug test.

The claim that a hair test cannot be tampered with has been shown to be debatable. One study has shown that THC does not readily deposit inside epithelial cells so it is possible for cosmetic and other forms of adulteration to reduce the amount of testable cannabinoids within a hair sample.

Legality, Ethics and Politics

The results of federally mandating drug testing were similar to the effects of simply extending to the trucking industry the right to perform drug tests, and it has been argued that the latter approach would have been as effective at lower cost.

Psychologist Tony Buon has criticized the use of workplace drug testing on a number of grounds, including:

1. Flawed Technology: The real world performance of testing is much lower than that claimed by its promoters. Buon suggest that tests are probably adequate for rehabilitation and treatment situations, possibly adequate for pre-employment situations, but not for dismissing employees.
2. Ethical Issues: Because of the fairly simple ways that an employee can invalidate the test, drug testing must be strictly monitored. This means that the specimen must be observed leaving the body. Many legal objections currently being raised in the courts about drug testing are pointing to legal requirements of prior notice, consent, due process, and cause.
3. Wrong focus: As has been shown with Employee Assistance Programs, the focus of management concern should be on work performance decline. Buon suggests effective management practices are an infinitely better approach to managing workplace alcohol and other drug issues.

Tony Buon has also reported by the CIPD as stating that "drug testing captures the stupid—experienced drug users know how to beat the tests".

United Kingdom

A study in 2004 by the Independent Inquiry into Drug Testing at Work found that attempts by employers to force employees to take drug tests could potentially be challenged as a violation of privacy under the Human Rights Act 1998 and Article 8 of the European Convention of Human Rights. However, this does not apply to industries where drug testing is a matter of personal and public safety or security rather than productivity.

United States

In consultation with Dr. Carlton Turner, President Ronald Reagan issued Executive Order 12564. In doing so, he instituted mandatory drug-testing for all safety-sensitive executive-level and civil-service Federal employees. This was challenged in the courts by the National Treasury Employees Union. In 1988, this challenge was considered by the US Supreme Court. A similar challenge resulted in the Court extending the drug-free workplace concept to the private sector. These decisions were then incorporated into the White House Drug Control Strategy directive issued by President George H.W. Bush in 1989. All defendants serving on federal probation or federal supervised release are required to submit to at least three drug tests. Failing a drug test can be construed as possession of a controlled substance, resulting in mandatory revocation and imprisonment.

There have been inconsistent evaluation results as to whether continued pretrial drug testing has beneficial effects.

Testing positive can lead to bail not being granted, or if bail has already been granted, to bail revocation or other sanctions. Arizona also adopted a law in 1987 authorizing mandatory drug testing of felony arrestees for the purpose of informing the pretrial release decision, and the District of Columbia has had a similar law since the 1970s. It has been argued that one of the problems with such testing is that there is often not enough time between the arrest and the bail decision to confirm positive results using GC/MS technology. It has also been argued that such testing potentially implicates the Fifth Amendment privilege against self-incrimination, the right to due process (including the prohibition against gathering evidence in a manner that shocks the conscience or constitutes outrageous government conduct), and the prohibition against unreasonable searches and seizures contained in the Fourth Amendment.

According to Henriksson, the anti-drug appeals of the Reagan administration "created an environment in which many employers felt compelled to implement drug testing programs because failure to do so might be perceived as condoning drug use. This fear was easily exploited by aggressive marketing and sales forces, who often overstated the value of testing and painted a bleak picture of the consequences of failing to use the drug testing product or service being offered." On March 10, 1986, the Commission on Organized Crime asked all U.S. companies to test employees for drug use. By 1987, nearly 25% of the Fortune 500 companies used drug tests.

According to an uncontrolled self-report study done by DATIA and Society for Human Resource Management in 2012 (sample of 6,000 randomly selected human resource professionals), human resource professionals reported the following results after implementing a drug testing program: 19% of companies reported a subjective increase in employee productivity, 16% reported a decrease in employee turnover (8% reported an increase), and unspecified percentages reported decreases in absenteeism and improvement of workers' compensation incidence rates.

According to US Chamber of Commerce 70% of all illicit drug users are employed. Some industries have high rates of employee drug use such as construction (12.8%), repair (11.1%), and hospitality (7.9-16.3%).

Australia

A person conducting a business or undertaking (PCBU—the new term that includes employers) has duties under the work health and safety (WHS) legislation to ensure a worker affected by alcohol or other drugs does not place themselves or other persons at risk of injury while at work. Workplace policies and prevention programs can help change the norms and culture around substance abuse.

All organisations—large and small—can benefit from an agreed policy on alcohol and drug misuse that applies to all workers. Such a policy should form part of an organisations overall health and safety management system. PCBUs are encouraged to establish a policy and procedure, in consultation with workers, to constructively manage alcohol and other drug related hazards in their workplace. A comprehensive workplace alcohol and other drug policy should apply to everyone in the workplace and include prevention, education, counselling and rehabilitation arrangements. In addition, the roles and responsibilities of managers and supervisors should be clearly outlined.

All Australian workplace drug testing must comply with Australian standard AS/NZS4308:2008.

In Victoria, roadside saliva tests detect drugs that contain:

- THC (Delta-9 tetrahydrocannabinol), the active component in cannabis.
- methamphetamine, which is found in drugs such as "speed", "base", "ice", and "crystal meth".
- MDMA (Methylenedioxymethamphetamine), which is known as ecstasy.

In February 2016 a New South Wales magistrate "acquitted a man who tested positive for cannabis". He had been arrested and charged after testing positive during a roadside drug test, despite not having smoked for nine days. He was relying on advice previously given to him by police.

Refusal

In the United States federal criminal system, refusing to take a drug test triggers an automatic revocation of probation or supervised release.

In Victoria, Australia the driver of the car has the option to refuse the drug test. Refusing to undergo a drug test or refusing to undergo a secondary drug test after the first one, triggers an automatic suspension and disqualification for a period of 2 years and a fine of AUD$1000. The second refusal triggers an automatic suspension and disqualification for a period of 4 years and an even larger fine.

Historical Cases

- In 1993 Meritorious Marine Sergeant Steve Steinmetz refused to submit to further drug screening on the grounds that it violated his 4th and 5th Amendment Rights against unwarranted search and self-incrimination. He was court-martialed and given a Bad Conduct Discharge from the United States Marine Corps in 1994 for refusing to obey a "lawful order". He was threatened with forced medical procedures to obtain a sample if he was imprisoned. Said Marine stated, "That won't happen". He was discharged without being imprisoned.
- In 2000, an Australian Mining Company South Blackwater Coal Ltd with 400 employees, imposed drug-testing procedures, and the trade unions advised their members to refuse to take the tests, partly because a positive result does not necessarily indicate present impairment; the workers were stood-down by the company without pay for a week.
- In 2003, sixteen members of the Chicago White Sox considered refusing to take a drug test, in hopes of making steroid testing mandatory.
- In 2006, Levy County, Florida, volunteer librarians resigned en masse rather than take drug tests.
- In 2010, Iranian super heavyweight class weightlifters refused to submit to a drug test authorized by the Iran Weightlifting League.

Doping Side-effects

The side effects of doping include:

S1 ANABOLIC AGENTS Anabolic Androgenic Steroids (AAS).

These are the substances that have both anabolic and androgenic properties. 'Anabolic' means 'tissue building' and 'androgenic' means 'masculinizing'. The anabolic properties may affect accelerated growth of muscles and bones while the androgenic properties may affect development of male reproductive system and secondary male sexual characteristics such as hairiness and deep voice. The anabolic androgenic steroids can be derived both endogenously (natural) as well as exogenously (synthetic).

After administration of anabolic androgenic steroids the formation of protein is promoted in genital organ, skin, skeleton and muscles. Athletes may be tempted to use anabolic androgenic steroids to improve their physical and physiological capacity to train and compete at highest level by reducing associated fatigues and recovery duration. In an impression to increase muscular power and strength these substances are sometimes taken by athletes involved in weightlifting, throwing and other sports involving strength parameters.

Side Effects of Anabolic Androgenic Steroids

The side effects associated with anabolic androgenic steroids are extremely serious and are divided into general, male specific and female specific.

General Side Effects

- Greasy skin and acne.
- Infertility.
- Hypertension.
- Liver and kidney dysfunction.
- Aggressive behaviour.
- Tumour.

Male Specific Effects

- Breast development.
- Testicular atrophy.
- Diminished male hormone production.
- Diminished sperm production.
- Impotence.
- Alopecia.
- Prostate cancer.

Female Specific Effects

- Male pattern hair growth and baldness.
- Menstruation disturbances.
- Decreased size of breast.
- Deeper voice (hoarseness).

Other Anabolic Agents

Other anabolic agents are substances which pharmacologically are not related to anabolic androgenic steroids, but may have the similar anabolic effect. This class of substances has been added in the WADA list of prohibited substances and methods because of clenbuterol and zeranol abuse in sports.

Side Effects of other Anabolic Agents

- Trembling.
- Restlessness, aggressive behavior.
- Anxiety.
- Arrhythmias.
- Muscle cramps.

S2 Hormones and Related Substances

Peptide and glycoprotein hormones are natural substances that act as 'messengers' within the human body and triggers the production of other hormones endogenously like testosterone and corticosteroids. The synthetic drugs like hCG, hGH, ACTH and EPO are known as analogues having similar effects to peptide hormones. Erythropoietin (EPO) hormone increases the number of red cells in blood and is used by athletes in endurance performances. Human growth hormones (hGH) are used by athletes for muscular strength. Human chorionic gonadotrophin (hCG) hormones are used by athletes to increase endogenous production of steroids specially to in an impression to improve the muscular strength. hCG is usually taken by those athletes who takes anabolic steroids to counteract the effects of testicular damage or as a masking agent. The use of synthetic gonadotrophin hormones by athletes stimulates ovulation in women and testosterone in men. Insulin may be illegally used in conjunction with anabolic steroids in an attempt to increase muscular strength. Adrenocorticotrophin (ACTH) hormone increases the level of endogenous corticosteroids in the blood and hence is taken by athletes in misconception to improve muscular strength.

Side Effects of EPO

- Increased viscosity of blood,
- Hypertension,
- Myocardial infarction,
- Cerebral infarction,
- Pulmonary embolism,
- Convulsions.

Side Effects of hGH

- Acromegaly (overgrowth of limbs),
- Soft tissues swelling,
- Abnormal growth of organs,
- Arthropathies (joint disorders),
- Diabetes mellitus.

Side Effects of hCG

- Menstrual disorders,
- Gynecomastia (breast development in males).

Side Effects of insulin

- Hypoglycaemia,
- Nausea,
- Drowsiness,
- Brain malfunctioning.

Side Effects of ACTH

- Insomnia,
- Hypertension,
- Diabetes mellitus,
- Stomach ulcers,
- Osteoporosis.

S3 BETA-2-AGONISTS

Beta-2-Agonists if taken into bloodstream are having anabolic effects and hence WADA prohibited the use of all Beta-2-Agonists by athletes with the exception of inhaled formoterol, salbutamol, salmeterol and terbutaline to treat and/or prevention of asthmatic athletes. An abbreviated therapeutic use exemption certificate is required for the use of inhaled Beta-2Agonists.

S4 Hormone Antagonists and Modulators

These substances may be illegally used by athletes to counteract undesirable side effects associated with anabolic steroid use such as gynecomastia.

Side Effects of Hormone Antagonists and Modulators:

- Hot flushes.
- Gastrointestinal disorders.
- Fluid retention.
- Venous thrombosis.

S5 Diuretics and other Masking Agents

Masking agents are substances that have the potential to impair the excretion of prohibited substances to conceal their presence in urine or other doping control samples or to increase haematological parameters.

S6 Stimulants

Stimulants are substances, which have a direct stimulating effect on the central nervous system. The stimulant increases the excitation of brain and spinal cord, cardiac output and rate of metabolism. The stimulants that are widely used in sports are amphetamine, cocaine and ephedrine. The players use these substances to attain the same effect as adrenalin, which is secreted naturally in human body. The stimulants may produce alertness, wakefulness and increased ability of concentration. These substances may develop the faculty to exercise strenuously or produce a decreased sensitivity to pain.

WADA has forbidden the use of stimulants in sports. Many cough and cold medications contain stimulants. One group of stimulants is the sympathomimetic amine of which ephedrine is an example. In lower doses these amines are often present in cold and hay fever medications and often these medications are easily available from pharmacies and retail outlets without the need of medical prescriptions. Thus such type of medications should be avoided by the athletes.

Side Effects of Stimulants

If an athlete after consuming stimulants performs under severe circumstances eg long periods and or in the heat, the athlete's body heats up intensively and due to influence of stimulants it may become difficult for the human body to cool down. The cardiovascular system and other vital organs also start malfunctioning by the use of stimulants and in some cases may lead to death. Other potential harmful effects of stimulants are listed below:

- Loss of appetite.
- Insomnia (loss of sleep).
- Euphoria.
- Hallucinations (Psychosis).
- Trembling.
- Restlessness, agitation, tenseness.
- Hypertension.
- Palpitation and heart rhythm disorders.
- Hyperthermia (increased body temperature).

S7 Narcotics

The narcotics prohibited in sports are those derived from morphine and its chemical and pharmacological analogues.

These substances act on central nervous system and reduce pain feeling. The use of narcotics causes a false sense of cure in an injured athlete that leads to ignorance of a potentially serious injury and risking further damage.

Side Effects of Narcotics

- Addiction.
- Loss of balance and coordination.
- Nausea and dizziness.
- Insomnia & depression.
- Decreased heart rate.

S8 Cannabinoid

Cannabinoid is psychoactive chemical. Marijuana, hashish and hashish oil are derived from cannabis plant. Prolonged use of cannabinoid may result in loss of motivation, decreased concentration, impaired memory and learning disability, respiratory diseases such as lung cancer, throat cancer and chronic bronchitis.

Side Effects of Cannabinoid

- Impaired balance and coordination.
- Loss of concentration.
- Increase in heart rate.
- Increased appetite.
- Drowsiness.
- Hallucination.

S9 Glucocorticosteroids

Glucocorticosteroids are prohibited in-competition when administered orally, rectally, intravenously or intramuscularly. Administration of glucocorticosteroids through these routes requires therapeutic use exemption certificate (TUE). All other routes including anal, aural, dermatological, inhalation, intra articular, nasal and ophthalmological require athletes to follow abbreviated therapeutic use exemption certificate (ATUE).

Side Effects of Glucocorticosteroids

- Fluid retention.
- Hyperglycaemia.
- Systemic infections.
- Musculoskeletal disorders.

P1 Alcohol

Alcohol is a central nervous system depressant which slows down the actions of the brain and body. Combining alcohol with other drugs can magnify the effects of alcohol or of the other drugs which can be dangerous in many circumstances.

Side Effects of Alcohol

- Impaired judgment.
- Loss of reflexes and muscular co-ordination.
- slurred speech.
- sleepiness and poor respiration.

P2 Beta Blockers

These drugs may be illegally used by athletes in precision sports requiring accuracy and steady limbs eg archery, shooting, modern pentathlon, luge, diving, bob sleigh, ski jumping and motor sports.

Side Effects of Beta Blockers

- Hypotension.
- Decreased heart rate.

M1 Enhancement of Oxygen Transfer

Blood doping may be illegally used to increase red blood cells in an attempt to improve the oxygen carrying capacity in endurance events.

Side Effects of Blood Doping

- Increased blood viscosity.
- Clotting susceptibility.
- Hypertension.
- Vasoconstriction.
- Kidney dysfunction.
- Risk of cardiac arrest, brain stroke and pulmonary embolism.

M2 Chemical and Physical Manipulation

Chemical and physical manipulations including catheterization without medical justification and masking agents are prohibited methods and should not be used by athletes.

Side Effects of Manipulations

Cystitis (bladder infection) and other dysfunctions and disorders depending upon the type of manipulation.

References

- Hoffman, Ronald; et al. (2009). Hematology : basic principles and practice (5th ed.). Philadelphia, PA: Churchill Livingstone/Elsevier. pp. Ch68. ISBN 0443067155
- Connor, James; Woolf, Jules; Mazanov, Jason (January 2013). "Would they dope? Revisiting the Goldman dilemma" (PDF). British Journal of Sports Medicine. 47 (11): 697–700. doi:10.1136/bjsports-2012-091826. PMID 23343717. Retrieved 15 July 2013

- Connor, James; Jason Mazanov (2009). "Would you dope? A general population test of the Goldman dilemma". British Journal of Sports Medicine. 43 (11): 871–872. doi:10.1136/bjsm.2009.057596. Archived from the original on 2 October 2013. Retrieved 15 July 2013
- Landy Justin F., Walco Daniel K., Bartels Daniel M. (2017). "What's Wrong with using Steroids? Exploring Whether and Why People Oppose the use of Performance Enhancing Drugs". Journal of Personality and Social Psychology. doi:10.1037/pspa0000089
- Joyner, MJ (Jun 2003). "VO2MAX, blood doping, and erythropoietin". British journal of sports medicine. 37 (3): 190–1. doi:10.1136/bjsm.37.3.190. PMC 1724644. PMID 12782539
- Staub, S.; et al. (2010). "Analysis of Hemoglobin-Based Oxygen Carriers by CE-UV'Vis and CE-ESI-TOF/MS". Electropheresis. 31: 1241–1247. doi:10.1002/elps.200900513

Permissions

All chapters in this book are published with permission under the Creative Commons Attribution Share Alike License or equivalent. Every chapter published in this book has been scrutinized by our experts. Their significance has been extensively debated. The topics covered herein carry significant information for a comprehensive understanding. They may even be implemented as practical applications or may be referred to as a beginning point for further studies.

We would like to thank the editorial team for lending their expertise to make the book truly unique. They have played a crucial role in the development of this book. Without their invaluable contributions this book wouldn't have been possible. They have made vital efforts to compile up to date information on the varied aspects of this subject to make this book a valuable addition to the collection of many professionals and students.

This book was conceptualized with the vision of imparting up-to-date and integrated information in this field. To ensure the same, a matchless editorial board was set up. Every individual on the board went through rigorous rounds of assessment to prove their worth. After which they invested a large part of their time researching and compiling the most relevant data for our readers.

The editorial board has been involved in producing this book since its inception. They have spent rigorous hours researching and exploring the diverse topics which have resulted in the successful publishing of this book. They have passed on their knowledge of decades through this book. To expedite this challenging task, the publisher supported the team at every step. A small team of assistant editors was also appointed to further simplify the editing procedure and attain best results for the readers.

Apart from the editorial board, the designing team has also invested a significant amount of their time in understanding the subject and creating the most relevant covers. They scrutinized every image to scout for the most suitable representation of the subject and create an appropriate cover for the book.

The publishing team has been an ardent support to the editorial, designing and production team. Their endless efforts to recruit the best for this project, has resulted in the accomplishment of this book. They are a veteran in the field of academics and their pool of knowledge is as vast as their experience in printing. Their expertise and guidance has proved useful at every step. Their uncompromising quality standards have made this book an exceptional effort. Their encouragement from time to time has been an inspiration for everyone.

The publisher and the editorial board hope that this book will prove to be a valuable piece of knowledge for students, practitioners and scholars across the globe.

Index

CPSIA information can be obtained
at www.ICGtesting.com
Printed in the USA
LVHW060907030122
707669LV00002B/397

9 781639 874057